Your Story Is Your Medicine

A Prescription for Healing in an Imperfect World

SHELLI STANGER NELSON, RN, BS

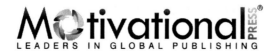

Published by Motivational Press, Inc.
1777 Aurora Road
Melbourne, Florida, 32935
www.MotivationalPress.com

Manufactured in the United States of America.

ISBN: 978-1-62865-310-6

CONTENTS

DEDICATION

This book is dedicated to my lifesavers: My brother Scott A. Stanger, Jason A. Bleistein, and "The Sweet One." And to all of those who are living the hour-to-hour challenges of diabetes; to all of those sitting on dialysis and waiting on a list; to those who have fought a good fight and lost; to all whose hopes yet spring eternal.

"Hold on, Baby hold on.
Your tomorrow's not the same as today."
– Written by Kerry Lingren, produced by Kansas 1980

ACKNOWLEDGMENTS

Thank you to the many people who had a hand, an eye, and ear invested in this work.

My heart holds exceptional gratitude for Rachael Freed of Life Legacies

And

Laurie Harper of Author Biz Consulting.

Additional heartfelt thanks to Nancy Stanger, Paul Strohm, and Louise Woehrle.

FOREWORD

IN JANUARY 2014, I MET WITH A SHAMANIC PRACTITIONER. I HAD limited previous exposure to this type of sacred work, but a trusted colleague suggested I try it to get some help with a particular issue. I scheduled a phone session.

During our conversation I nonchalantly sat on the loveseat in our living room. Outside, Minnesota had just experienced a day of wintery weather. The clouds, heavy and the color of dove wings, capped the dome of the sky. Crystallized ice and snow clung to the branches of the trees on the wooded lot of our suburban home. When the wind blew, the branches shook with a sudden shiver, scattering pieces of frozen snow-diamonds against the windows. My foot, covered in a well-worn slipper, made contemplative circles on the top of the oak coffee table, a long-ago Christmas gift hand-made by my brother, Scott. It was a day of ordinary events: supper simmered in a pot on the stove, the dog gnawed on a raw beef bone at my side, insistent e-mails sounded as they entered my in-box. But it wasn't an ordinary day at all. Without knowing anything about me, the practitioner said, "Your medicine is your story. You need to tell your story."

The practitioner offered me her wisdom about my medicine, which was not the reason for my call, and I was silent. When we were finished talking, I hung up the phone, got up from the loveseat, and thought, "Well okay. It's time for me to tell my story."

And then I did nothing. Well, nothing to begin to write the story, that is. I returned to working as an RN in a cardiac unit, returned to seeing therapy and bio-energy healing clients in my private practice, and returned to the school of bio-energy healing and transpersonal psychology I own and operate with my husband. I went back to the things I was doing every day: writing newsletters for the academy, shooting videos for YouTube, doing laundry, making meals, working out at the gym, and fighting to make it through a Minnesota winter of epic frigidity.

Although my spirit-self understood that the message uttered by the Shamanic practitioner held immeasurable wisdom, I didn't heed the advice—at least not right away. "I'm too busy to write a book," was my first thought. Then the voices in my head convinced me that while I could write newsletters and little stories, I could *not* write a whole book. The idea of a book felt like navigating an ocean liner down the Mississippi River. My story was too big and I felt too small to write it.

Then three months later, in April, I experienced another. . . health crisis? Blessing? Lying in bed one late afternoon, my body tense with unanswered questions, my future laced with uncertainty, I returned to the words I'd heard on the loveseat: "Your medicine is your story." And in that very moment I felt a rush of hope that seemed to emanate from my soul, to fill my body. As it did, a forgotten part of me was ignited. In that instant I felt a sensation inside my flesh, in my bones, which reminded me of how I felt with my first kiss. Immense clarity rippled through me that was so explosive, it burst through the ends of my hair. I fully understood the message. The time had arrived for me to take action.

This book is my medicine, medicine for me, and hopefully medicine for you.

This book is my story. People who are mentioned in this book could have their own story about particular events or general times. Their stories may be different than my story. Yet each story is true because all events are relative to the observer. I've summoned all the courage I possess in order for me to write openly and honestly. The word, "courage" comes from the Latin word, "cor" which means "heart." When it was first used in the English language it meant to tell the story of who you are with your whole heart. And so it is with the intention of providing myself with my own medicine that I begin my story.

And so it is.

Shelli Stanger Nelson

INTRODUCTION

THIS BOOK IS ABOUT MANY THINGS: IT'S ABOUT MY UNCOMMON MEDICAL conditions. It's about how I learned to integrate devastation into my life in a real way that honors both the insanity of the experiences and the tenacity of the spirit. It's about how blessings and recovery can be birthed from nearly every tragedy. But mostly, it's about healing.

When I hear the word "healing" I feel judgment and embarrassment, but primarily, I feel hope. My judgment arises from attending workshops and meeting many people who vigorously throw the word "healing" around. Yet in my experience, few people offer substantive treatments or ideas that lead to meaningful and abiding change for me.

The idea of healing also evokes feelings of embarrassment. I'm a scientifically trained nurse with sophisticated education. My western, linear mind says science and medicine are the interventions leading to health and vitality. Yet I own a successful healing practice and operate a licensed school of healing. I can feel embarrassed when I talk with my medical colleagues about this side of my professional work. Sometimes I stammer for words as I stand at the nurse's desk, trying to convince another clinician or physician that a cancer or heart patient may benefit from discovering the emotional and spiritual aspects of his or her disease. Or that I really truly can run energy from my hands that affects the physical body in ways that have resulted in reversal of thyroid deficiency, for example, or has changed the pictures seen on an MRI of a shredded ligament to a normal one after a handful of thirty-minute treatments.

More than anything, though, the idea of healing fills me with hope. Beyond the doubtful doctors and well-meaning practitioners lies a potential for resolution, restoration, salvation, restitution, and peace that can all be found in *healing*.

What exactly does it mean to heal, be healed, and to experience healing?

Through my own healing experiences, I've learned that healing is a journey rather than a destination. Healing takes many forms, each one essential and necessary. We heal physically; our cells, flesh, bones and blood get healthier. We heal emotionally; our relationships, our injured feelings, our emotions about being sick or our emotions about all the let-downs, heart breaks, trampled dreams, and our own overbearing, idiotic, self-absorbed and self-abandonment reactions to life's events get healthier. We heal mentally; our thoughts and judgments about past or present situations, the self, and others get healthier. When we heal mentally, our opinions and beliefs get healthier. And we heal spiritually; our union with a Divine Source greater than the self is strengthened and the connection becomes healthier and morphs from an external process to a tangible, internal sensation.

When we address all the aspects found in every trauma, whether that's a physical injury or illness or a mental, emotional or spiritual breakdown, we are becoming healthy. "Health" comes from the Anglo Saxon word meaning "whole." It doesn't mean absence of disease, which is how most western societies define health. When we heal, we become whole.

Physical healing may or may not include eradication of diseases, physical pain, or restoration of a broken body. As someone who has had to manage a life filled with multiple illnesses, excruciating pain, and the possibility that my diseases could end my life, the idea of anything short of a "cure" can seem like failure. When it comes to illnesses and conditions that may limit my longevity or force me to live with physical restrictions, what I want is a cure, not to make peace with disease or, God forbid, death. For many years I held a belief that "cure" was the only meaningful, and necessary, healing. I didn't give a damn about making peace, understanding my chronic illnesses, or accepting the slow and steady destruction of my body. It's part of human nature to want to survive and to live free of illnesses or emotional upheaval. And yet once I was able to drop the demand that I be granted my every wish about physical health, my life experience truly improved. Not from a bullshit, "I'm okay, let's make lemonade from lemons" platitude, but authentically, genuinely, less painful and less intolerable. Believe me, if it weren't so, I'd shout it to the world that all of this healing talk is a bunch of euphoric bull designed by people who dance around with garlands in their hair and have no appreciation for the often bitter reality of existence.

In order to heal emotionally, we must be willing to feel and express our full range of emotions: about illness, loss, relationships, and other traumas. Healing emotionally also means we are willing and able to express our love, excitement, and enthusiasm. Healing emotionally doesn't imply reaching some sort of nirvana wherein we only feel pleasant emotions. On the contrary, it implies understanding one's emotions and being able to express them in an appropriate manner. After we have healed emotionally we are able to contain our emotions when necessary and we express them robustly when the situation calls for such expression. We stop using emotional states as a definition of the self. "This is just the way I am. I'm not a happy person." I know that part of my emotional healing, which could be the case for you, too, was to first be able to fully express my rage and fury over the outrageous, unthinkable happenings that had become my life story. I also needed to learn that it was safe for me to express my happiness and euphoria in an appropriate way without being afraid of being shamed or ridiculed.

When we are healing mentally, we are working toward greater understanding of our opinions, our beliefs, and our judgments of self and others that limit our perspective and set up biases and self-righteousness. We are figuring out where and why we first created these ideas. Eventually, we are able to open enough to invite these thoughts to change and evolve. Our opinions and beliefs morph from exclusivity to inclusivity.

These inclusive opinions, habits and beliefs do not negate our inalienable rights as Divine human beings. Rather, we experience a shift that maintains our fundamental rights without using a hierarchical belief system that impedes the same rights of all people. Our beliefs, thoughts and opinions become healthier.

When we heal spiritually we are aiming for one goal: to recognize and feel the co-mingling between the self and the source of all creation, whatever name any person may ascribe to that entity.

It is a part of our birthright to heal. Physiologically, our bodies are designed to sustain injuries and illnesses, and heal from them. Physical healing is often the easy part. We come down with chicken pox or the flu and we get over it. But we don't "get over" a missing limb, violence, or many other catastrophic traumas. I don't believe we get over blindness or the death of a child. Instead of "getting over" these things, we can learn to integrate the event and all that resulted from it into the rest of our life. Each of us heals uniquely from these intrusions. One of the goals is learning how to turn down pain that screams like a siren so that we can, once again, allow other aspects of life to have a prominent voice.

It is a common misunderstanding that burying trauma is an effective means of healing. It does not heal, but it is a useful coping skill until we are ready for authentic healing. In the process of denial, the hurtful experiences remain in the subconscious and in the body's cellular memory. Over an extended period of time, denial can make matters worse. Repressed anger can lead to long-standing grievances and resentment. Unexpressed fear becomes anxiety, which can lead to even more debilitating conditions. Withholding sadness can become depression or can lead to social isolation. As an energy medicine professional, I also know that suppressed emotions over an extended period affect the physical body and lead to real illness.

Each of us heals at our own speed. How quickly we heal depends on many factors, including internal resources. Sometimes we need to stay in the safety of denial until we have sufficient internal fortitude to open the story for healing. Sometimes we need to remain in a state of anger or rage for a long time. The beginning phase of healing often requires the individual to stay in the "story." We need to tell the events of our stories over and over as we understand them, before it's time to move on to the next step of healing. In fact, if we try to rush the process, clamor toward complete optimism, redemption, and forgiveness, we're denying our real emotions and opinions, and cannot achieve authentic healing. We cannot heal what we refuse to admit about ourselves, others, and the real circumstances of our lives.

Our stories can be our medicine, as long as we are willing to believe that lessons, gifts and blessings abide beneath the distress of the story.

It took me a long time to be willing and able to accept this as a truth, rather than dismiss it as an abstract concept or as airy-fairy wishful thinking. Doing the deep work of my own healing has allowed me to experience life with optimism, exuberance and love, despite circumstances of the past or potential difficulties that may cause me suffering in the future. If you are willing to use your story as your medicine, to face what is deep within you, then you can live life with strength in the midst of fear, with courage when you feel weak, and with hope when life is treacherous.

Mine is a very unusual, ordinary life--unusual in that I've experienced events that most people never encounter in a lifetime and ordinary in that I'm just an average person. Ordinary people aren't unremarkable. They are doing amazing, holy, and sacred work every day; they just don't realize it. Holy and sacred is the work of the sister who is at her brother's hospice bed in his home, making meals, watching his strong frame shrivel before her eyes until he is nearly transparent. Remarkable is the daughter who, after twelve years of being estranged from her mother, one day picks up the phone and with a trembling voice says, "I can't carry the burden of being apart from you any longer."

We all have important stories to tell, whether it be to our private journals, to our brother living in Calcutta, or to our loved ones or strangers. This commonality provides us companionship as we search for a safe haven in which to reveal the truth of our stories. Each person's story is valuable and those stories can provide healing for the self as well as others.

My hope is that reading this book helps you find your holy work, your eternal courage, your magnificent nature and that you too, allow your story to be your medicine.

"Stories have to be told or they die, and when they die, we can't remember who we are or why we're here."
Sue Monk Kidd

"We all live inside our stories."
Salman Rushdie

"As we tell our stories we often discover the divinity that is present in our lives."
Rabbi Laura Geller

"There's a story behind everything.
How a picture got on a wall. How a scar got on your face.
Sometimes the stories are simple, and sometimes they are
hard and heartbreaking."

Mitch Albom

"After nourishment, shelter and companionship,
stories are the thing we need most in the world."

Philip Pullman

Chapter One

THE SWEETNESS

It's May, 1973. I'm ten years old, running barefoot through the open yards that surround the homes on the block where I live. Most of the twenty-four kids who also live on the street run and shout with me in jubilant pleasure. It's Saturday – the best day! I've watched morning cartoons in my jammies and eaten my favorite breakfast made by my mom: waffles with maple syrup and little sausages. As I run, I feel my skinned knees burning from yesterday when some of us were drinking root beer floats while playing on the swing set. I fell off my swing, but saved my frosty glass of creamy delight! Today we're playing a sweaty game of kick ball in the afternoon sunshine. Someone's mother shouts to us, "Lemonade and cookies!" and we dash over to rest in the ever-present comfort found in the food our moms provide.

I guzzle down a glass of lemonade and help myself to the oatmeal cookies. I frantically drink another glass of the sweet liquid and still one more. I can't get enough to drink.

Soon it's close to dinnertime and the gang of kids slowly dwindles. At home, I turn on the garden hose and drink feverishly. Then I find an empty half–gallon orange juice bottle and fill it with the chilly water. Taking the bottle with me to the back steps, I sit and gulp down every last drop. I'm incredibly thirsty. For the past few weeks, no matter how much I drank, my thirst was never quenched.

Mom approaches me from around the house. She's carrying a yellow, plastic laundry basket loaded with clothes she's taken down from the lines. "Shelli! Are you drinking again?" she asks me with surprise. I feel embarrassed. She's noticed how much I've been drinking lately and has already made other comments. I feel like I might be doing something bad. I shyly reply, "I'm so thirsty. The water just isn't wet enough." Mom eyes me suspiciously as she proceeds past me on the steps with her load of laundry and goes inside to get dinner on the table.

The next morning Mom brings home a small, blue tablet from work that's wrapped in a piece of foil. Mom works the night shift on the pediatrics unit as a nurse's aide. She asks me to catch my urine in a plastic container. Mom uses an eyedropper and puts some of it into a soda can mixed with some water and drops in the blue tablet. I'm standing at the kitchen sink with her, standing on my tip-toes, straining as I watch the blue tablet make the liquid fizz and begin to turn colors. When the fizzing stops, the liquid inside the can is orange. "What does that mean?" I ask. Tossing the can into the trash, she replies, "It means you might have diabetes."

I have no idea what diabetes is or what having it implies. I'm scared.

I've been to the hospital many times already. I accidently overdosed on medicine twice before I was four years old; one time I took my Grandmother's sleeping pills when I was barely two. I still remember the ambulance ride, the needles in my arms and my shrill screams when I was put in a bed with a net over it as Mom and Dad left the hospital ward. When I was in first grade I accidently stuck a wire abacus down my throat. When I yanked it out, I tore my throat open. The people at the hospital stuck another needle in my arm before I went to surgery to repair the damage. Last year I fell and broke my arm in three spots. The broken bone protruded hideously out of my skin at one place. I shrieked in pain when the hospital people moved my arm around to take X-Rays. More needles; they hurt. I don't know what diabetes means, but I sure hope needles aren't involved.

Mom tells me if I have diabetes I will have to quit eating anything with sugar. I get a sinking feeling in my heart. *No sugar?* I think, recalling all the play and treats at everyone's house. *What else is there?*

Beyond my apparent tendency to be accident-prone, the first decade of my life was average, ordinary and mostly benign. My whole family and everything we did was Minnesota average. My father, Gene, worked as a barber, snipping and brushing, chitchatting with his all-male clientele. He's the son of an average milkman who married an average first generation German woman who completed the eighth grade and then worked full–time until she was eighty–five years old. My mother, Karen, worked for fifty years, first as a nursing assistant and then at a clerical job in the local hospital. She is the daughter of a simple man who delivered oil to houses and farms in the 1940's and 1950's. And her own mother was an average woman who taught Sunday school, knitted sweaters, and worked at the dime store.

My parents were nineteen years old when they married and started our family. I was born thirteen months after my only sibling, Scott.

Our German heritage informed us that there is one important thing in life: work—housework, schoolwork, job work, lawn work and so on. Understanding this one important element in life made living simple: Just do your work and everything will be fine. I eased through each day with little difficulty. I did the work expected of me, followed the rules as best I could, and looked forward with equanimity to each day's vibrant beginning and restful ending.

Based on the first ten years of my life, it appeared as if my childhood would be ordinary and similar to all the other kids I knew. I liked my easy, predictable, stress-free life. I could count on grilled hamburgers every summer and picnics at a redwood table in our backyard. I knew each spring I'd get a new swimsuit cover-up hand-made by my mother. I knew each July we would vacation in our car, driving across the country to National Parks where we would hike on trails and pose for pictures at scenic overlooks. Each autumn, I'd walk to the same elementary school with the same kids from our neighborhood. I loved school: The learning, the social atmosphere, the smell of pencils and paste and lined notebook paper. I anticipated the same hot lunch menu year after year and was comforted by the familiar, homemade hot dinner rolls smothered in butter served with turkey and gravy over mashed potatoes. We laughed our way through Christmas at Gramma and Grampa Stanger's house. Each year the same frosted cakes, cookies, potato salad, meatballs, and Christmas pudding appeared on the white tablecloth festooned with red poinsettias. My parents kept us safe and happy. We played board games on the floor of our living room, and watched movies together on the only television set in our house. I swung vigorously on the neighbor's swing, skated on the ice rink at the park, rolled up snowmen in our yard, and looked forward to the tender snuggle of my warm bed in my room, with the pink dotted–Swiss wallpaper Mom and I picked out together.

I had few concerns in my childhood. There were few decisions to make in this predictable, carefree existence. I loved my easy life that seemed normal, constant, and required only age-appropriate responsibilities and understanding. Life remained easy and sweet until the spring of 1973.

I'm sitting with my mother in our busy pediatrician's office. I'm wearing my new blue bumper tennies. Kids are waiting for their annual exams or their vaccinations but I'm there for a different reason. Last week Mom put the blue tablet in the soda can holding my urine and it turned orange. I'm here to find out if I have diabetes. I still don't understand what diabetes is other than I know it means no more candy bars, ice cream, or Mom's homemade desserts. I also somehow know that diabetes will change my life forever, and not in a good way. I spent last night alone in my room, trying to sleep. As I softly gazed at the Holly Hobby sticker I had put on my closet door and my doll sitting on a shelf, bewildering thoughts cluttered my mind, thoughts too complicated for a ten-year old. As I wait for my name to be called in the doctor's office, I wish I could run away, back to my safe bedroom, the kick ball game, the lemonade stand, and oatmeal cookies.

Mom and I are escorted to an exam room and we wait. Inside I feel like birds are loose under my ribs but I'm not going to admit it. My body language tells a different story: "I'm a warrior and not afraid of anything in this office." Fear is something I'm unwilling, and afraid, to show. I simply refuse to look weak or bothered by anyone or anything. Being afraid shows weakness and showing weakness means vulnerability, which I believe can lead to more trouble, like someone making fun of me or hurting me in my exposed state. "How are you doing?" Mom asks me while we wait. "Fine," I say matter-of-factly. I decide my tennies need re-tying.

A nurse brings a shiny tray into the exam room. The items on the tray include all sorts of scary looking materials, even the gauze, which I know means blood.

Silently the nurse tears the paper off of a flat square package revealing a small corner of a thick, pointed piece of surgical steel. Without saying a word, she rams it into the tip of my middle finger. It feels like I've been stung by a hornet. I resist crying or even flinching. I pretend it doesn't hurt. I sit with my knees pressed tightly together; my teeth are clenched and I'm holding my breath, hoping the event will pass more quickly. The nurse sticks the end of a clear, glass tube on the end of my finger and I watch the brilliant red line of my blood rise up and fill the tube. The nurse efficiently gathers up her supplies and leaves. Mom and I wait.

After a century of minutes, Dr. Schauffhausen comes in. She is a tall, reed-like woman who has a Lauren Bacall voice and a cool, patrician face. She's wearing a mint green dress under her white lab coat. I wish she'd take off that white coat and turn into a safe sales lady at the department store. "Well, her sugar is 499," she says to my Mom. "Let's run her in," the lanky lab coat says looking only at my mother. Poof! She turns and is gone.

My head is reeling. My mouth is slightly agape and my eyes look to my mother's as I fidget with my small fingers in my lap and twist the toes of my blue tennies into the floor. *Run me in where?* I wonder, confusion churning in my head. My small heart is thumping in my chest.

What's happening? Where am I going? My mind is a whirlwind of unanswered questions. Mom is getting up. Everything's moving too fast. Sitting frozen in a chair too big for my body, I look longingly up to my mother's face, searching for any indication about my demise. "Do I have it?" is all I ask. "Yes, you do," is all she says.

In oppressive silence, we make our way through the noisy waiting room where kids are still playing with brightly colored plastic cars and rocking rubber–headed baby dolls. They're staying and I'm leaving. We get into our car and drive directly to the hospital. Here my education about how I will live for the rest of my life will begin.

The nature of my required work will instantly change. At ten years of age, I will be expected to inject my leg with a needle to give myself insulin. I will learn how to handle a syringe and how to draw up the insulin I need from two bottles. I'll be expected to be certain I have the precise amount each time. I will learn to measure my sugar level by counting drops of water and urine into a test tube and dropping a blue tablet into it four times every day.

I will learn about food restrictions and how to be diabetic. I will learn that the sweetness and ease of living is gone, slipping from my hand as quietly and easily as releasing a bird's feather.

It will be a very, very long time before I will recapture any sense of ease in life again. And even then, I will never, *ever, be the same.*

THE HEALING

Although it was decades ago, my memory of that time is as vivid as if it were happening right now. It was only recently that I realized the magnitude of what happened back then. On May 10, 1973, I lost my childhood: my sweet, easy, ordinary life. I lost the freedom to simply be a child. I lost my child-sized work and daily concerns. The loss devastated me.

Being forced to leave behind the life I loved left me feeling cheated. I felt forgotten. I also felt my distress was invisible and I had to grow up with a moment's notice. I didn't want to live an existence wherein I had to be restrained. I didn't want to be logical and reasonable. I mourned that I had to surround myself with scary needles and testing equipment. I was angry, but more than that, despondent, that I was now different from everyone else. None of the other twenty-four kids on my block had to pee in a cup every four hours. No one else had to stand in the bathroom alone, using an eyedropper to count pee and water into a test-tube and drop a blue tablet into it. No one else in our house was required to sit alone at the kitchen table on a cold morning, the darkness of night still thick outside the single window, and tear open alcohol swabs and stick a needle in their leg or arm. Everyone else could eat the hot lunch at school and drink root beer floats.

Everyone else kept right on with their lives; every other kid kept being a kid, but I had to be accountable.

I wanted my child-work to be making my bed and sweeping the floor. I wanted my work to focus on learning how to paint my nails and curl my hair. I did these things. But every hour I was also monitoring for dangerous symptoms. I couldn't just scamper to the breakfast table and gulp down some apple juice and eat what the rest of the family was eating. While everyone else ate caramel rolls or a stack of pancakes doused in thick, delicious maple syrup, I ate Kix cereal with skim milk or a single pancake with watery, horrible tasting saccharine syrup substitute. I had to think about what I was eating. I had to keep log-books and recordings all day, every day.

The loss was much bigger than the food–although that was hard. All of the "fun" events focused around food. It wasn't just sugary treats, but regular food as well: a glaze made with pineapple juice or bread and butter. Beyond that, the center of all joyful gatherings was the dessert, the treats. And even more important than the sweet snacks was food--the central highlight of any social gathering or commemorative occasion. I couldn't have the gooey indulgences that were specifically designed to reward accomplishments, heighten celebrations, and provide comfort. But any food, even carrot sticks, negatively influenced my blood sugar and within hours of eating, I'd feel sick and achy. While the rest of the crowd indulged, I sat separate, sipping Diet Rite cola or eating something not nearly as glamorous. It was lonely and I felt sad and jealous of the laughter and satisfaction I saw in other people's faces as sugar hit their brains.

Since I couldn't have the desserts, nor the majority of the rest of the food, my experience of the event was not joyful. Everyone I knew ate pastries and sugar to feel good. Not only did I have to give up the food, but I also lost the fun and anticipated climax wrapped within it.

One of my healing moments was when I realized how much I had been conditioned to view food and desserts as the core highlight of any celebration. Everyone I knew ate pastries and baked goods in order to feel good. For me there was no Christmas, there was no reward or fun or happiness without sugar and the food associated with the event. Because the events were no longer fun, I might as well have stayed home. I had unconsciously carried this hidden belief with me my whole life.

Revealing this hidden belief allowed me to release the repressed emotions that still clung to me and were still influencing my thoughts and behaviors-even though I didn't realize they were. When I became aware that I had felt as though I were an outsider and believed that I couldn't have fun at social gatherings like everyone else, I was a bit stunned. I learned that my discomfort at parties and holidays was linked to this belief, and was not because I was a curmudgeon who'd rather be home and left alone to pout. My inner dialogue was now able to change!

Before my healing moment, I found celebrations to be occasions that left me feeling unhappy rather than filling me with spontaneous laughter. Sometimes I even felt judgmental and angry watching celebrants joking and enjoying themselves while I stewed in unhappiness that I couldn't explain. I began to believe I was unfriendly and cantankerous. I devalued celebrations as being a meaningful part of life. Not surprisingly, people picked up my unspoken messages and I was seldom invited to parties, which pushed me deeper into feeling like an outsider and amped up my sadness. Sounds pretty screwy, right? But this is what happens to all of us: we hold a belief. We project this belief into the world and the world responds similarly, thus proving our distorted image as truth rather than a result of our own projections.

After my realization, I was able to form different beliefs about what made social occasions fun. I learned that the person I am today is not the ten-year-old who wanted caramel apples. I learned to enjoy the people, or the conversation. With the truth of my real sadness revealed and the hidden belief released, I now experience celebrations in a whole new way and I have dropped the abusive self-talk that overshadowed my true essence.

This is an example of how finding and healing buried beliefs and their associated emotions can have a dramatic impact on one's life experience. Being able to laugh and feel the thrill of parties may not seem like an extraordinary achievement. But my newfound awareness of how I came to feel disengaged was astounding. It is a normal part of human relationship to want to be part of a group and to enjoy celebratory moments. For me, this healing allows me to have a more fulfilling experience of life. We all desire and deserve to feel happy and to be able to experience life as a member of a group. Consider that you may have images or beliefs about life that you are totally unaware of that prohibit you from feeling the full measure of pleasurable moments. Every belief we hold that impedes us from fully enjoying life has its root in our past. By discovering the origin of these limiting beliefs, we can change them, if it is our desire to do so. When we do, we can become more content.

I had a lot of mourning and unexpressed grief over all of this loss but I repressed the mourning. As a child I followed the rules and did what was expected of me. I felt my sadness, but as a child I didn't understand it and I didn't have words to express it. My defenses against grief and fear instructed me to "soldier on," be strong, move ahead. Over time, this repressed mourning grew, but I was unaware of it. Instead of recognizing the mourning, I grew angry. It was safer for me to say I was pissed than it was to say I was sad. Sad people were weak and a bother to be around. Angry people were strong and were a force to be reckoned with. If someone wanted to duel with me, I was primed and ready for the ensuing battle. It felt great to work off my rage. But the combat did nothing to touch my true emotion of sadness and the feeling of being prohibited from experiencing the same gaiety and blissful memory of a shared affair. While others sat with half-lidded eyes, oohing over the sublime comfort derived from food, I looked on, longing to join them and to feel what they were feeling. In my child mind it felt like everyone was getting a gift at the party except for me. What's worse is that I felt I was supposed to be fine with this arrangement, but I wasn't!

The moment my childhood was interrupted by the insult of diabetes I developed a coping strategy; the impulse to run away when faced with a situation that could alter the course of my life. This defensive desire to run continued to grip me for much of my life, and I can still feel the urge to do so if the threat I'm facing feels especially dire.

For decades I felt an internal discontentment simmering below the surface. It hindered my ability to relax, to feel at peace, even on an ordinary day. I felt slightly anxious most of the time. I felt an insatiable internal craving that frustrated and perplexed me. No matter what I did to try to fulfill this need, to soothe the craving, or to feel at peace, it didn't work.

I finally realized what I craved was a return to my average, ordinary, and simple existence that had been abruptly taken from me. The sorrow of that loss lay alive in my mind and in my body. I needed an emotional healing that would also help my physical body.

From the moment I left the doctor's office with the diagnosis of diabetes, my life became complex. As the years went on, ease and simplicity eroded until even the basic act of writing my own name was challenging. I was astonished when I understood that my defense strategy to run was not about running away from these real complexities and struggles. It was about running back to a time when living was easy, simple, and sweet, back to a time when I could just be. Now I understand that when I want to run back to being a child, it's not that I'm childish or irresponsible, it's that I'm remembering the sadness of my interrupted childhood.

When I finally understood what the insatiable craving was about, I felt a tremendous relief. This was the healing. When I could name the source of my discontentment and my defense to run away, my suppressed emotions released. That release lifted the internal persistent craving, the tension and discontentment, and I was more able to enjoy the present moment of life without feeling restless and agitated. The understanding gave me clarity. I understood that the craving of childhood could not be fulfilled today. The emotions I feel about the loss of an easy, uncomplicated life remain, but now they are contained rather than buried.

Forty-three years later, I sometimes still weep for that lost little girl and the burning wish for a life that is trouble-free. Even "normal" stressors that all responsible adults experience can occasionally nudge me into my wish, and I think that's normal. Today I can reach that tipping point because of some fractional, inconsequential happening, like burning my toast. I know that's because I'm already carrying a hefty load. So today the toast burns, I cry and I know my tears aren't about the toast. It's a relief to know that I'm really weeping for the lost freedom of being a child who so desperately longed for a simple, fun life that she saw everyone around her enjoying. And for the adult I've become who also wishes that her daily stressors were average and mainstream.

Because of the interruption of my childhood, I feel passionate and compassion about infringements on children's rights and childhood illnesses. Every child deserves the childhood I started with: to feel safe and protected at home, to have predictability that offers comfort, and to be free from worries, responsibilities, and pressures that are too complex for a child's mind. Diseases, abuse, neglect are abstract ideas that confuse children; they are not equipped to make sense of them. Besides, childhood is brief: It ought to be filled with the blissfulness of simplicity, of imagination, and of play. Childhood ought to implicitly provide a body and spirit that is whole. This is my hope, and I believe if we put energy into the things we hope for, those hopes can become a reality instead of remaining a dream.

As I healed the sorrow of my abbreviated childhood, I learned that although I can't redo those years, I can comfort the little one who still lives inside me. I can recognize her sadness and instead of asking her to grow up or move on, I can hold her close in my fully grown consciousness and wrap her in my strong adult heart.

One of the luckiest things in life that can happen, I think, is to have a happy childhood.

– Agatha Christie

In my soul, I am still that small child who did not care about anything else but the beautiful colors of a rainbow.

– Papiha Ghosh

Chapter Two

THE VILLAIN, THE FRAUD, AND GOD

IT'S 1998. I'M IN MY BED; MY HUSBAND IS SLEEPING BESIDE ME. IT'S THE middle of the night when I wake. I'm completely dripping in sweat. My pajamas and the sheets are sopping wet. I'm weak, shaky, confused. I know I need something, something to make me feel better, but what? I know I'm in a dangerous situation. The experience is familiar and the symptoms quite distinct. I stagger down the short hallway in the pitch darkness. I bump into the corner of the hall where it turns into the front foyer and become totally lost in my own home. Nothing is familiar, even the floor and the banister I'm now holding are disorienting rather than anchoring. Clueless as to where I am, I can't move an inch. My mind is reaching–reaching for something familiar, something solid for it to land on to help me figure out where I am and what I need to do.

My head bobbles loosely on my shoulders. My eyes are half-open heavy slits, vacantly staring at the pitch-dark floor. *Concentrate*, I say to myself, *Just stand here and think*. My thoughts move in slow-motion, like the sound of voices under water. I think about the thoughts, think about why I'm having the thoughts, think about how the thoughts feel moving in my sluggish brain, and finally, think about what to do about the thoughts.

With maximal effort, I shuffle into the kitchen where I slump against the pantry doors. *What now?* is my next thought and the whole thinking process begins anew. Standing there in my kitchen, now naked because I've peeled off the drenched nightgown, I find a sliver of coherency that allows me to locate the knob on the pantry door and understand that it needs to be opened. *Now what?* I stand wavering as the sweat continues to run in rivers down my face, off my nose, and cascades down my torso and legs to my feet where I stand in a puddle of accumulating perspiration. I'm freezing deep in my bones. My entire body trembles. My body is too much for me to keep upright, so I slump into the pantry resting on my forearms, my head hanging and my mouth drooling. *Think, think. Why are you here?* I grope in the pantry - maybe my hand will find what I need. As I fumble around in the pantry my hand lands on a stack of juice boxes that I drink when my blood sugar is too low. A flicker of coherency reaches my brain when I touch the familiar object. One is usually enough to bring me back to safety. Now I drink three of them.

I wait. No change. I drink another, and wait some more. I lean my forehead on the pantry shelves. I can't move. The symptoms worsen. My orientation is fading with each passing second. I'm dizzy; the room spins and my thoughts are disconnected, muddy syllables trapped in my brain. Suddenly I'm hit with impending doom. *I'm going to die tonight.*

I'm in the terror for several minutes, wondering what I'll feel when I take my final breath and my heart stops. Then I hear a different voice. My thoughts and words instantaneously connect and I say out loud, *It's only death. It's like walking through a doorway. You've done this before. It will be nice, actually.* I make my way back down the hall and deliberately and peacefully lie down in my bed beside my husband and wait with acceptance for death to come. I fall asleep. Morning comes, just like it has so many times before.

What am I supposed to say about a disease I've had for over forty years that savagely stole my life, my dreams, by the time I was twenty-three? How can I put that down in a few pages? The last thing I wanted to do in my life was to re-visit the history of my pain and suffering. I wanted to stay in the comfortable place I find myself today, after all the crawling on the floor and screaming in the bathroom and sobbing in hospital rooms. I didn't want to think about the story, and I certainly didn't want to immerse myself in the story. I wanted to skip right to the healing and the gifts.

Yet as I opened myself to a past that I experienced as decades of hourly torment, I discovered how much of that suffering still lay dormant in me. I still had memories stuck in my body that ached for release and relief. The memory was very much alive and closer to the surface than I wanted to believe. It gave me even greater appreciation for the importance of doing my work–again.

I had to find confidence that the more healed parts of myself could do this work; that this part of me would be able to hold the broken one as I began to write my story that would serve as my medicine.

"Diabetes is a disease of the blood vessels," Dr. John Baumgartner, my prior endocrinologist and past president of the American Diabetes Association, said in his lecture to my nursing class in 1984. "Because it's a disease of the blood vessels there's no place in the body unaffected by diabetes." Little did I know he was forecasting much of my future.

In the beginning, at least for me as a ten-year-old, diabetes was just about losing out on walks to the corner store for a Popsicle on a sweltering summer day, or having to forgo apple pie fresh out of the oven after school. In the beginning, diabetes was only about regimented meal times, sitting in the nurse's office eating five Ritz crackers and a piece of packaged cheese while the rest of the 6th graders were playing dodge-ball in the gym. Or watching happy kids at the lunchroom table drinking their chocolate milk and smacking their lips on banana cake, while I ate canned pears swimming in water from a plastic dish. It was about feeling like an outsider who wasn't welcome to join the fun.

In all honesty, the restrictions of food and the accompanying sense of being outside the group never changed. In time, however, the uncomfortable, internal physical sensations, the long-term destruction of my body, and the emotional impact of daily coping became the seemingly insurmountable problems.

Diabetes is much more than the loss of cake and pie.

I'm in my new blue and white spring pajamas. Jo Graff, one of the pediatric RN's that works with my mom, gave them to me as a gift for my trip to the hospital. I'm sitting on the side of my hospital bed. I'm ten years old. I've been in the pediatrics unit for nine days now, learning how to manage diabetes; learning the diet I will be required to follow for the rest of my life; and learning how to inject myself with insulin that has been harvested from cows and pigs.

My nurse, Val Bang, comes into my room, wearing a white uniform and cap and a gentle smile. I'd rather see my mother; she worked last night, but she's been sent to the family lounge. I'm told I can see her afterward. I'm going to give myself my first injection.

I draw up the insulin, two different types, while Nurse Val watches to be sure I have it exact -even one tiny bit over or under can make me sick. I pull up the leg of my pajamas. Delaying the inevitable, I rub the tender skin of my leg for a long time. I feel butterflies in my stomach and the sensation makes me even more scared. My throat is tight. I want to cry, but I don't want Val to know I'm afraid. She might tell my mom.

Tearing open the alcohol pad, I wince; the odor is noxious and I already associate the smell with fear and pain. I wipe my skin and pinch the tissue of my leg with my left hand over and over, as if to find a spot that has no pain receptors. I sit for many minutes staring at the point of the needle poised millimeters above my skin.

"Push it in," Val says.

I touch my skin with the point of the needle. It's sharp. I cave to my fear and cry.

"Push, push," she coaches me.

I try. I'm scared. I want my mom. I want to go home. I want to go anywhere that is far away from now. Slowly, I work the needle in, advancing it by tiny lengths. It is taking me over ten minutes to advance the needle. "I can't do it," I finally say through my inconsolable tears.

"There's no such word as 'can't'," Val retorts.

Still staring at the needle half way into my leg, I say, "Yes there is; you can't put toothpaste back in the tube." She doesn't argue with me.

Eventually, I get the needle all the way in, push the plunger and successfully complete the first of hundreds of thousands of injections. In time, when my blood sugar will be too high, I will crave the needle like a heroin addict. Or I'll loathe the sight of the orange-capped syringe, throwing it violently to the floor in a fit of rage and grief.

My eleventh birthday arrived a couple of weeks after I was discharged from the hospital. With that event I learned the first thorny truth about diabetes: food is a part of everyday life, every social gathering, and no matter what the food, it is a diabetic's nemesis.

During my ten days of hospital "internment," I was instructed from an orange book covered with a cartoon face. This manual explained how I was to weigh every ounce of meat on a postal scale and measure every portion of every bit of food in a tin measuring cup. I learned I would eat every meal within thirty minutes of a prescribed time. I was to count out vanilla wafers, or saltine crackers, or weigh a chunk of cheese on a kitchen postal scale and count out twelve medium-sized grapes–not ten or sixteen–exactly twelve every time. I was to do this for every single morsel of food for every single meal for the rest of my living days, forever and ever! What a set up for failure.

It wasn't bad at first. It was like a new talent or learning how to play a musical instrument. My new diagnosis and specialized skill of self-injections made me special. But once I had demonstrated my unique ability to my friends, the curiosity dwindled and they moved on. Soon I grew weary of the restrictions and the regimentation of diabetes. My family kept their sugary desserts, their malted milks, and second helpings of blueberry muffins while I sprinkled saccharin from a pink packet on corn flakes and avoided making eye contact with the brownies sitting on the countertop. They all lathered their burgers with barbeque sauce and ate fruit salad dotted with colored mini-marshmallows topped with whipped cream, while I ate my burger dry and poked at the little dish of fresh fruit beside my plate. It seemed to me they didn't even notice that I was isolated and enduring a lonely struggle of solitary misery.

The shelves of our home were stocked with packages of indulgences that I was supposed to ignore and instead eat half a banana or a sliver of plain angel food cake. It was hard to languish over a saccharin sweetened soda when the television showed mountainsides of happy, hand-holding people singing "I'd like to buy the world a Coke," and the Coke was right in our refrigerator.

I did the best I could for much of the day. I counted and measured; then at night, or when alone, I sneaked the glorious pleasure of homemade peanut butter cookies or chugged Hawaiian Punch reserved for Scott from the fridge. The next day I'd try again: measure, count, measure, count. I ate the special desserts Mom made for me: vanilla wafers crumbled atop crushed pineapple and tried to feel indulged and satiated. It didn't work. When no one was watching, I went back for the gingerbread cake and whipped cream that everyone else had eaten with that night's dinner.

I concluded that I was a hopeless, weak loser.

I just couldn't do it. And the more I couldn't, the more I pretended it was easy. And the more I pretended, the deeper I fell into a bottomless chasm of shameful self-loathing and a profound internal belief that I was a miserable failure, liar, and an embarrassment.

Dad smiled, gleaming at me when family members were present, their concerned faces asking if it wasn't tempting for me to have the desserts and ice cream that were in the house. "Oh, she does great; she knows her diet and doesn't have a bit of trouble, do you?" Dad would proudly say as a statement, not a question. *"Lie,"* I could hear my inner self saying, *You have to lie. If you're not strong enough, you're weak, and then you're bad and a disappointment.* The familiar sensation of Raggedy Ann guts was back. My heart raced with trepidation as though I had just teetered on the edge of something. *Be careful!* A voice inside me screamed, *Don't disappoint him. Say whatever is necessary to make him proud.*

Standing there, my family members watching me, my memory flashed to all the times Dad pointed at the cookies, Pop Tarts, and donuts. "These aren't for you. No fail." His expectation engulfed our little kitchen. "No fail, no fail."

"Oh, no, it's really not hard. I just know I have to, that's all, so I do it," I'd say with an air of fearlessness. Instead of admitting I needed help, and dealing with the consequence of failing Dad, I pretended to be confident and responsible beyond my years. I interpreted the messages from my dad to mean I shouldn't need help, that needing help was unacceptable. I felt that needing help implied I was "helpless." Helpless people were a pain in the ass, a burden, and could be kicked out of the group for being inconsiderate of others' valuable energy and more important needs.

I lived with diabetes for thirty-five years. I call it the thirty-five-year war. It was a living hell on an hourly basis. Diabetes ruled every aspect of my life. The disease was aggressive. Even when I became an adult and had my own home that wasn't stocked with things I shouldn't eat and could comply more easily with the dietary guidelines, maintaining steady blood sugars was never easy for me.

Sugar is an essential component for the function of the brain; too little sugar and the brain simply turns off, like the time in my kitchen when I searched the pantry. These times were generally accompanied with a sense of impending doom that was profoundly real.

It's Halloween night. My husband and I are watching *Schindler's List* on video. Suddenly I begin to feel disoriented. I recognize the distinct and familiar symptoms of hypoglycemia, a blood sugar level that's too low. The sounds from the TV are distorted. My brain is fogging up. I snatch up some of the trick-or-treat candies and shove them into my mouth. I wait for the fog to lift. No change. Fear rising, I eat more of the candy. The doom comes, but it comes so quickly, I'm unable to tell my husband I need help. I'm now having bizarre thoughts. In a split second, rapidly firing scenes of my entire life show up on my mind-screen. Real occurrences that are vivid, yet totally insignificant; occurrences that wouldn't readily stay in one's memory, like my neighbor lady from when I was eight years old smiling at me as she shook her bathroom rugs or two cars pulling into our driveway one winter afternoon. I don't have enough functioning brain cells to respond to the signals alarming my body to get help immediately. I'm no longer a part of reality, lying on my family room sofa watching a movie; I'm now in the movie. I'm one of those helpless people soon to be tortured or murdered in the Holocaust. I appear totally normal from the outside, but I'm actually swiftly heading toward a diabetic coma.

I'm in a world of sounds that are distinct, sensations that are vivid. I clearly hear the mournful violin music of *Schindler's List*. My husband is kneeling on the floor beside the sofa on which I lay, but I don't recognize him to be my husband. My malfunctioning brain is convinced he is the Nazi Doctor of Death, Dr. Mengele, who is going to do a lethal experiment on me. He has hold of my arm and is aggressively attempting to inject something into my vein that I believe will kill me.

My head lolls back and forth; I'm in abject terror. I'm searching for something to say or do to save myself from this sinister plot, to fend off my assailant. "No. No. No." My muscles have all the strength of an April leaf. I lie in a semi-comatose state. The dark recesses of my brain urge me, *"Do something. You're not a Jew. Save yourself. Fight. If he gets that needle in, it will be all over for you."*

"I'm not a Jew, I'm not a Jew," slurs from my barely functional tongue. I feebly fight and attempt to take back my arm. I'm sure the syringe he has contains some sort of nerve toxin or equally inhumane substance, not the injectable sugar that will save my life. "Stay quiet. Hold still," he instructs me in a firm, whispered voice. He becomes more deliberate and aggressive with me, insisting I surrender to his scheme. His forcefulness makes me more terrified. He's bigger and stronger than me. I have little strength. I believe I'm about to be murdered. How can I rescue myself?

I'm lying in a pool of sweat. My sweater and pants cling to me in a chokehold. I believe the Nazi has tied me down or others have arrived to help with my murder. I'm hysterical inside, but I have little power in my body. I know I need to get up, run, fight, scream, but I'm paralyzed. I'm slipping deeper into semi-consciousness and I believe it's because I've been injected with the evil serum. My voice is barely audible as I mutter over and over, "I'm not a Jew; I'm not a Jew." I'm unresponsive. My husband can finally get the needle into my vein and depresses the plunger. He sits back on his heels and waits, all the while watching me, hoping. Time passes.

I begin to become aware of myself in the room. I recognize the movie; I can feel my damp clothes. My husband sees I'm coming back. No ambulance needed this time. Seeing that I'm out of danger, he recaps the needle of the spent syringe and says with a smirk, "I'm not a *Jew? What the hell*?"

Of course my husband had no idea my sugar-deprived brain had created a completely different reality that was vividly real in my world. I explained what my mind had created. We laughed hysterically. The adrenaline in both of us needed escape. Instead of collapsing to the floor sobbing, we laughed. Behind the safety our laughter provided, we both knew the truth. Had I been alone, I might not be alive at this moment. This wouldn't be the last time we would navigate the fine line between life and death with diabetes.

I was never sure when these low blood sugar times would hit. At one moment I'm talking on the phone, alert, oriented, and the next moment I'm sliding off an icy cliff. I can't say how many times my husband saved my life. It got to the point where he was afraid to leave me alone. On vacation he left me to unpack in our bed and breakfast and returned twenty minutes later with a bottle of soda and a book to find me slumped on the bed delirious. At night he would reach over in our bed and find me in a clammy mess, unable to wake me up. He'd go to the garage to do something after dinner while I'd be doing the dishes. When he came back inside an hour later, I'd be zombie-like wandering around our kitchen, talking nonsense.

I rarely found middle-ground in managing blood sugars, despite gallant efforts. Either I was sucking down juice boxes and walking in a fog, or my blood sugars were too high. High blood sugars also made my brain murky. I felt lethargic with aching muscles. I felt nauseated and crabby. My emotions changed. The physical symptoms made me irritable and frustrated. My body was being destroyed and I had little ability to do anything to change it.

I'm on a bike ride with my husband. I stop every thirty minutes to make sure my blood sugar is within a tolerable range. We finish a picnic lunch at a beautiful waterfall along a parkway. My blood test reveals that the chef's salad I ate with an apple and some crackers has caused my blood sugar to spike to four times normal, despite the insulin I had taken and the rigorous exercise. We pull over on the bike trail. Other people are walking by, biking, and roller blading. Balancing our tandem bike between our legs, my husband draws up a small amount of insulin. I offer him the vein in my arm and create a make-shift tourniquet with my hand. He shoots me up with the IV insulin. A mother pushing her kid in a stroller looks at us from the corner of her eye and walks hastily past us.

We're about to go into a comedy club with friends. I test my sugar and find it's excessively high. We find a dark corner. Standing there, I push up my sleeve and my husband sticks a needle in my vein, hoping no one has questions.

We're on vacation and about to eat breakfast at an outdoor tropical restaurant. As usual, I test my sugar at the table: too high, even though it was at a good level an hour ago when I woke up. Sitting there at our table, we do the IV insulin routine so I can eat. Even so, I feel like crap and I'm miserable another day with fluctuating blood chemistries that make it impossible to "get away," even on a vacation.

In a twenty-four hour period of time, every single day, my body went through this up and down cascade of constantly changing glucose levels. Diabetes consumed me, literally and figuratively. Everything focused on what my blood sugar level was. It determined whether or not I was going to be able to eat, and if I could engage in any physical activity, like walking through a store. Even sex depended on what my blood sugar reading was. Some people brush their teeth or put on lingerie in anticipation of a romantic moment. I tested my blood sugar and gave my husband the report about whether we were a go for that night. I tested my blood sugars with a finger prick eight to fourteen times every day. The disease was aggressive and unpredictable.

I counted every carbohydrate I ate once the doctors realized this was the best method for tracking how much insulin to give. I wore an insulin pump on the outside of my body, attached by a thin IV-like tube that was inserted into my tissue. That didn't work either, and I felt like I was held prisoner, except I had no idea what my crime had been. Giving insulin intravenously isn't standard procedure. My diabetes doctor instructed me to give small doses of IV insulin when my blood glucose levels were excessive. I had to try to get the sugar in a somewhat safer range very quickly.

I was constantly hyper-vigilant for any miniscule physical change I experienced. On the one hand I was fearful that I would find myself half-witted with a falling sugar level that I couldn't save myself from. On the other hand, I often found my sugar levels so high I needed IV insulin just to get it into a somewhat safer range.

It was common for my sugar level to change significantly in only thirty or sixty minutes. I needed to be on alert at all times. Some people didn't understand how critically dangerous my condition was. Once when I was at a retreat one of the instructors thought I was being too vigilant and unnecessarily concerned. She suggested, "Why don't you just move like a reed in the water?" I wanted to tie the reed around her neck and toss *her out to sea*!

Despite the fact that all of this was happening on a perpetual basis, I worked, went to plays, hosted parties, cleaned the house, and chose to live a daily life like everyone lives. I would venture to guess that while people saw me testing my sugar and giving myself insulin, most people didn't know that while I was carrying on a conversation of great importance I was simultaneously sensing and interpreting every nuance in my body, moment to moment. Other than my husband, and maybe Mom, no one knew how hideous life with diabetes was for me, because I didn't talk about it. I was not going to be an energy-draining nuisance who needed emotional support and compassionate understanding. "No fail," rang through my brain. "It's no big deal." Even in my desperation, I negated my suffering.

There were many, many days and nights when I cried until I was completely drained. During the day, my friends, co-workers, and family saw me carry on as though my life was not all that different from theirs. And many a night I lay on the bed or on the floor of the bathroom, begging, pleading, sobbing to God to help me. Urgently, I beseeched whatever or whoever was out there to hear my pitiful call for mercy. There was simply never any rest. I was physically and emotionally exhausted. As the decades dragged on, the daily fight wore me out. I felt as if my spirit was pulverized to ash.

It's autumn in 2006. The trees in our wooded neighborhood are russet and crimson, gold and indigo. Millions of acorns are falling from the enormous, old oak that graces the front of our home; its beautiful branches stretch around our house like the arms of a mother inviting her children into them. In the air, the pungent scent of flowers turning to seed, and drying leaves and grasses float with an absence of effort. Squirrels work industriously; birds eat ferociously; geese fly purposefully, and the earth gives bountifully. For the past weeks I've tried to enjoy life and the brilliance of all that autumn brings with it in Minnesota, but I can't. I'm trapped in a daily deluge of tests, giving myself insulin, and trying to get my blood sugar to respond.

I'm lying on the floor of my treatment room. I've spent the better part of the last hour imploring God for help, for relief, not even for a cure, just a damn break! I'm bawling like a toddler, as I have so many times before, caught in hopeless anguish. My muscles ache and are cramping with the influx of excessive potassium caused by the equally excessive amount of sugar in my blood. My tongue, lips, and hands are tingling and sensitive; my heart is racing. "Please, I'm begging you, help me. Give me some signal that you are hearing me." The response I hear is cold, still, silent. I feel alone and utterly abandoned by The Divine.

On that day and countless other days I desperately spoke to what seemed like a heartless and callous Creator, asking for forgiveness for whatever I had done or didn't do. I groveled shamelessly on my knees for healing. I bargained, begged, and cried until snot ran down my lip and my body broke. I was a fraud; I was not a warrior and didn't want to be. Diabetes was killing me and I knew it. I couldn't do it anymore. I was totally empty and my faith was disappearing. How could there be a God when all this was happening? And if there was a God, why were my prayers unheard?

I clearly didn't matter to the Divine. I was being dragged into the pit of hell and God knew it. If I were important, He, She, It, would respond, send an angel, save me from the endless physical and emotional torment and the erosion of my body and spirit. If I mattered, there would be a sign, a change, a miracle. It would get better. Or better yet, be gone. I mean, miracles are supposed to happen, right? "Ask and you shall receive," right? Well, here I am, asking. Silence.

Anger replaced my desperation. Faith was a sham, a trick, a big fricking hoax. I was being laughed at by invisible spiritual perpetrators. God was a villain, a liar, a trickster. God was worth no more to me than the idiot doctors in their air-conditioned offices wearing their $2,000 Armani suits. The doctors sat referring to a damn computer print-out of my sugar readings of the last three months and offered me their pre-packaged advice that wasn't worth the paper it was written on. After my allotted ten minutes of time, the doctor would move on to the next room in the hallway of waiting patients and I'd be alone, again.

"Doctors and clinics receive financing according to the performance of their diabetic patients," Dr. Baumgartner said to the students at my school of healing in 2012. They don't get paid for digging in the trenches or being compassionate.

I was engaged in a hopelessly repeating nightmare of falling from a skyscraper, never hitting the ground or feeling safe, and then finding myself at the edge of the rooftop again, slipping over the side. Doctors weren't saving me. And much to my dismay, it appeared, neither was God.

Have you ever felt abandoned by God? Have you ever felt you were doomed to carry your suffering into eternity? You, like me at that time, might be thinking, *Healing and forgiveness isn't even on my radar; I'm still trying to have a single thought that isn't wrought with torment.* If that's how it is for you, that's okay. It took me a long time to accept that healing and forgiveness were possible. I wrote earlier that healing takes place on its own schedule and is dependent upon many factors. One is how much internal reserve a person has. Initially the injurious event depletes all our energy, because it's often all-consuming. Healing, forgiveness, and understanding cannot be birthed while we are struggling just to keep our nostrils above the water. Don't rush yourself! Don't force the process. If you're raging inside, admit it, claim it, accept it. If you're terrified or gripped with grief, let it be so. And if it's been too long, too many years of treading water, consider the possibility that healing and forgiveness could have a place at your table.

An early step in healing is to admit to yourself, and perhaps to someone else, that a piece of your heart is missing, a section of your soul is crooked. Most likely we know our life is out of order. One thing we are unaware of is that we are attached to the trauma, unwittingly hooked because the idea of healing and forgiveness seems outlandish, an insult to our justified anger, our normal fear, or our defensible judgments. At this time it's all right to say, "I'm pissed - I'm terrified - I've been robbed and cheated and I don't see any reason to feel differently." We can't stay in this mind-set forever, though, if we want to recover from our let downs or tragedies, whichever is the case. I've revealed my own sorrow, and now I ask you, "What is it that cries for healing in your story? What physical affliction, emotional struggle, or past or present offense brings you to your knees in the deepest hours of the night? What are the voices in your story that lament incessantly for understanding, forgiveness, and reprieve?" I've been transparent not only for the healing of my story, but to inspire you to look deeply within the stories of your life to discover the possibility of your own resurrection.

At this point in my story, my daily torment was feeling that I was a failure and thus, deserving of the destruction of my body. I held a belief that I would never escape from the whirlpool of continual dangerous events with diabetes that toyed carelessly with my life. I could not leave my life behind and take a vacation. What is the perpetual torment you live with that you wish to run from, but can't? I felt as though I was trapped in a net that not only tied me down, but choked me and got larger and tighter the more I thrashed for freedom. What is it that you've wrestled with your entire life, or for the past decade, that you can't escape? Like me, I'm sure you've tried every conceivable way to manage your problem, to regain control, and even to hide the fact that you're hurting and need help.

What is the loss you grieve on a daily basis? What events play unendingly in your mind as you go about your daily life? Like me, is there something you mourn daily, but your sense of pride, or your fear of being seen as weak or a burden, prevent you from reaching out for support?

Our troubles don't need to be all-consuming disasters in order for us to have legitimate need for healing and understanding. Our common disappointments and simple sadness are also worthy of a healing process. Any time our ability to have carefree, loving thoughts and a happy life is over-shadowed, we deserve some healing time. Too often we think, *This is so trivial compared to the troubles of others.* While this is a nice way to put things into perspective, it also minimizes our real experiences. We all deserve to have our experiences of both ecstasy and despair validated. Contrary to the popular platitude, it really *is* okay to complain if we have no shoes, even though someone else has no feet! Are there issues in your story that won't kill you, won't ruin your life, but leave a dark cloud over you just the same?

Sometimes we refuse communion with others because we believe that talking about our story is worthless and will only accelerate our turmoil. We can be so distraught or angry that we believe the notion of healing would be insulting and merely placating. It's normal to want a cure for our suffering rather than communion. At these times we say, "Why bother? Screw it." We don't want to move like a reed in the water, nor to make peace with God, nor find acceptance. We want nothing to do with anything that diminishes or takes away our self-righteousness and habit of complaining. When I was in this place, I held on to my insistent outrage, even though it kept me stuck in my unhappiness, and that's not where I wanted to be.

Have you locked yourself into an illusory room of isolation during the day and only come out of the dark when no one is watching? Has your heart been so desecrated that you are a prisoner to your demand that nothing short of a perfect life will ease your agony? What part of your story seizes you in a grip of regret so unbearable you fall to the floor and become a supplicant to the Holy? We can become so tied up in our trauma that it's easy to believe God is testing us, all the while holding our salvation in a locked vault. We can become so adamant that we get what it is we demand, that we push away the help being offered. We say, "No" to everything – even things we know could be beneficial.

This reaction is normal for a period of time. If that's where you are, no one is going to force you to change your mind. In fact, the more you're pushed, the more you might dig your heels in. Accept your no and your refusal, but own it. Admit that you're being stubborn and you don't want to be talked out of your misery yet. Honor the pain and the perceived injustices in your story. You'll know it's time for healing when you cannot carry the burden of your anguish any longer. When that time arrives, it is neither too late nor too early; it is your precise, right time.

THE HEALING

Diabetes taught me one of the most important lessons of my life: self-forgiveness. Self-forgiveness is the most challenging sort of forgiveness, self-admonishment the most destructive insult.

The disgrace I felt about my inability to comply with my diet in my childhood home plagued me into my adulthood. The punitive voice inside me chided and harassed me constantly, instructing me that I "should have" been able to resist temptation, have more self-control, and been stronger. It told me I deserved all the future destruction of my body. As I healed, I learned that diabetes is a set-up for failure. People who were diagnosed at the time I was were often dead in less than forty years, no matter the level of compliance.

The lesson of self-forgiveness expanded. I learned to forgive myself for things I'd done and later wished I hadn't; and to forgive myself for things I didn't do that I wish I had. Once I was able to experience internal redemption, I was able to extend more forgiveness and compassion to others as well.

As I healed the self-loathing part of me, I learned that I had been charged with a job that was too much for me to handle at a young age. I realized that I deserved to have more help with this challenge, but more than that, I learned that it was okay to need help. Even as an adult, I saw how often I refused to ask for help with anything. I realized I was stuck in a double bind that made me believe if people loved me, they would instinctively know what I want and give it to me without my having to ask. And on the other hand, if I didn't ask, no one would offer. It's *my* responsibility to ask for what I need. I had to come to terms with the truth that I have legitimate needs as a human being. Sometimes my needs can be met quickly, and other times I might have to ask several times and multiple people before finding the right person and time that can accommodate me.

For decades, I thought that if I were forceful with my disease I would develop greater authority over it, and believed my disease would somehow be tamed. I wrongly concluded that there were two options when facing challenges: fight and win, or, relax and die. The truth was that I very well might have died if I wasn't on alert, but I didn't need to fight with my disease; I needed to work *with it* by finding middle-ground. Middle-ground was a concept I wasn't familiar with. Fighting with it was exhausting me and the exhaustion was just as debilitating and destructive as the fight.

As I lay in my healing room that autumn day when I thought God wasn't hearing me, I eventually heard a voice in my head. At the same time it felt like the voice was outside of me, drifting in as I began to focus on the trees outside and the sound of the dying leaves falling without strife to the earth, *Don't try to kill it or it will get bigger. It's alive, too, and wants to live.*

What I learned that afternoon was one way I could find middle ground. I was fighting with a disease inside me, but I treated it as though it were not a part of me. I finally found a place where I didn't need to fight with it, but simply be vigilant and respect its impact on my life. I had to come to terms with the fact that it actually was *my* disease. When I treated it like it wasn't a part of me, I wasted a lot of energy being angry at it, feeling hostile toward it. When I owned that it was my disease, I felt compassion–compassion for me.

I learned that fighting, "superiority," and aggression, only gives an illusion of authority. I was able to recognize how much *willfulness* I relied on. Once I realized what I was doing, I was able to adjust my thinking and changed my disposition from willfulness to *willingness*. When I was willful, I wanted what I wanted, no matter the consequence. In my willfulness I was aggressive rather than assertive. Following the aggressive push and desperation of my will and the associated emotions of outrage that often accompanied it, I became so depleted that I would submit and collapse. It seemed I was split between two extremes. Then I became aware of a third place: that of middle ground, a state of willingness rather than willfulness. I became willing to tolerate what was present in my life, be it diabetes, external challenges, or my human limitations.

Since I had little past experience of finding or living in a reality where middle ground existed, it took me many attempts to reach balance. I often swung like a pendulum, not realizing how I ought to behave or feel, living life from the middle. With continual practice, I mastered a narrowing range where I find myself today. In this delicate place of willingness, aggression becomes acceptance and submission becomes compromise. In this middle ground state of being, I became willing to be open to more possibilities, one of which was the idea of surrendering the fight and surrendering the demand that I be in control.

Surrender was chillingly terrifying. I resisted it as though I were fighting for my life. The idea of surrender had always meant "I give up." I imagined white flags and being taken hostage, dragged away in chains and shackled at the feet with no escape possible. Surrender meant failure.

I discovered that surrender had little to do with failing or losing, or being subjected to the fanciful whims of others. Rather, it meant allowing a greater plan to emerge. In surrender, I am relieved of the necessity of knowing the answers and instead, can welcome a greater wisdom to take over. My limited, human brain doesn't possess all the wisdom pulsing through the universe. In the space of surrender, my human mind can hear what Spirit is saying to me. Answers came to me that were previously indiscernible and the search for justification of my victimhood. And in this expanded field of limitless possibilities where everything is possible, nothing is necessary. There is no need to fight or crawl, because there is no battle. There is no need to plead or collapse because there is no adversary.

It is then I am able to taste the sweetness of life and move like a reed in the water.

Ultimately, I surrendered to my powerlessness. A small part of me wanted to believe I was all-powerful and could dictate what events would be allowed in my life. I found a greater experience of authentic power by accepting that, in fact, I'm mostly not in control of anything. In this state of surrendering to my powerlessness, I found peace. I fell into the gentle and compassionate place where my demands were suspended.

When I began to live from this state of being, I found my indelible power. It is through accepting myself as a human with human limitation that I become limitless. When I no longer fight for control, I have freedom. In accepting my fragility, I am strong.

And so it is.

The truth is that our finest moments are most likely to occur when we are feeling deeply uncomfortable, unhappy, or unfulfilled. For it is only in such moments, propelled by our discomfort, that we are likely to step out of our ruts and start searching for different ways or truer answers.

M. Scott Peck

Nothing splendid has ever been achieved except by those who dared believe that something inside of them was superior to circumstances.

Bruce Barton

Life is a series of experiences, each one of which makes us bigger, even though it is hard to realize this. For the world was built to develop character, and we must learn that the setbacks and griefs which we endure help us in our marching onward.

Henry Ford

Chapter Three

FROM OUT OF THE BLUE

I'M FOURTEEN YEARS OLD, LOUNGING ON A TATTERED HANDMADE QUILT spread across shaded grass beneath a tree that's likely centuries old. I'm in the city park of a small farming town in Iowa. It's 1976– the bicentennial 4th of July weekend. I'm here for my annual summer visit to stay with relatives on their farm. The thermometer on the post beside the bank reads 101 degrees. I'm wearing faded, hip hugger jeans, a yellow and white spaghetti strap shirt and my Medic Alert bracelet dangles from my left wrist, the back inscribed with, "diabetes."

I'm carefully watching four boys, one of whom is carrying a yellow shirt draped over his shoulders and has a birthmark on his upper arm. His skin is richly tanned like cream in coffee, he has dark, curly hair, strong arms, and a cleft chin. I'm literally being carried away by the sight of him. I can't take my eyes, or my thoughts off of him. I study every move he makes. He is the single most gorgeous creature I've ever seen. Inside I feel things I've never felt before. I'm falling in love for the first time.

Tom is kind and polite with a gentleness that is endearing. He smiles at me with the tenderness of a butterfly landing on a daisy. Tom is different than other boys I know. His nature is gentle, his energy calm and steady, and he treats me as though I'm a fragile being who deserves tenderness. All of this encourages me to relax, even though when he looks into my eyes it feels as though I'll fall over where I stand. I feel I can trust him, something that isn't easy for me to do. He's funny and says such sweet things to me; I have to turn my eyes down in shyness.

If there is love at first sight, this is it.

We spent every moment together during my visit that summer. I felt I had found my best friend, a lost part of myself I didn't know was missing. My annual two–week visit with my relatives ended, and I returned home. We wrote to one another all summer, expressing dreams, thoughts, love, and our feelings of heartache because we were apart.

It was beautiful, magical, and exhilarating. There is no feeling that surpasses first love.

No one could have predicted what would transpire over the next twenty years based on a glimpse across the park, but then, isn't that just how our unusual, ordinary lives all happen? A nothing moment ignites a movement and shifts the tectonic plates of the soul. In that immeasurable unit of time, a permanent path is created. The story is now marked with a signpost reading, "I went this way."

Tom and I spent the next nine years in and out of relationship. Every year or so, we managed to see one another. Whenever we were together, we felt the same feelings of Eros and love. But distance was always a strike against us.

Our lives diverged. I enrolled in nursing school and eventually became engaged to Mike, a guy I had dated for many years, and Tom went to college and eventually joined the Air Force. Although we were moving on with what were separate lives, we were always in contact by phone or letter. In late November of 1984, I had second thoughts about my engagement. I called Tom, who was stationed in Denver with the Air Force. He encouraged me to come to Denver to ski, and to think about what I wanted to do.

I was a senior in nursing school, preparing to graduate in June. I was looking ahead to how I wanted the next stage of my life to unfold. Now that I wasn't convinced I would marry Mike, my options were changing.

It quickly became clear as we prepared for my January trip that neither of us needed to figure anything out; we were destined for a relationship that was more than casual. Tom and I decided I'd take my Nursing Board exams in Minnesota as well as Colorado and I'd move to Denver to be with him after my June graduation. Although we'd spent nine years in love and in some sort of relationship, we'd never been together for more than a week at a time. Clearly we would need to experience being together day-to-day, with its excitement and monotony, to know if marriage was right for us.

My mother was thrilled; she felt confident that Tom could handle my high- spirited passion for life, as well as the medical issues we all knew would be present with diabetes. She also knew how much I loved him from the first moment we met. In general, Tom was just a terrific guy that any mother would want her daughter to marry. He was self-directed, strong but gentle, funny and confident. At twenty-five he had already begun a sound plan that would lead to a successful life and livelihood.

It's January 1985. I'm eagerly anticipating my upcoming trip to visit Tom in Colorado during my winter break from nursing school. I'm in my bedroom looking at the pink, dotted Swiss wallpaper talking with Tom on the phone.

"I have an idea where you should look for a job," Tom says through a smile. "Okay, where?" I ask, smiling back at him, my heart in a suspended state of joy to hear his voice in my ear. "Amsterdam!" he says with enthusiasm.

I'm confused. Looking now at the falling snow outside my bedroom window I think, "Where in Iowa is Amsterdam?" I'm certain he's telling me he's moving back to Iowa.

"Where's Amsterdam?" I ask innocently. Laughing in his ever-present, slow, sexy drawl he says, "Baby, Amsterdam. Holland. The Netherlands. The country."

I'm crestfallen. Tom has received orders from the Air Force that he is being transferred overseas in May for a three-year tour. The plan we just conceived for me to work in Colorado as a nurse while we decide if marriage is right for us is gone. He's leaving. The idea that I could look for a job in Holland isn't realistic; I can't go with Tom as his girlfriend-we would probably need to be married. I'm sick to my stomach thinking he could decide to go to Europe without me, and so is my mother.

"Don't worry, baby, it will all work out," Tom, in his confidence, reassures me.

Two weeks later I'm sitting cross-legged at the dining table in Tom's Colorado condo. Wearing jeans and a white midriff shirt on which is written *Royal Gorge, Colorado*, I'm studying for my nursing boards. Tom comes through the front door wearing his Air Force uniform and a look of determination on his face. Looking at him on the other side of the room, I wonder what the problem is.

"Screw it, we're just gonna get married. There's no way to do it other than that," he says.

I could have cared less that we needed to get married right away! Moving to another country was way more than what I had planned, but if I did it with Tom, I'd move to hell wearing a dress doused in gasoline.

Tom left for Europe in May and we planned our wedding for late September, 1985. I was drunk with happiness at the thought of it all. I methodically crossed off each day on a calendar, my excitement building as more and more expired days accumulated.

I'm wearing a white wedding dress, the cathedral-length train trails behind me for an eternity. Regal trumpet music plays as I walk down the center aisle on my father's arm carrying two dozen pink roses in my hand. Candlelight fills the stone church with a soft glow as rain sprinkles down outside. At the altar, Tom stands at attention. He watches me coming down the aisle and we hold each other's gaze. My heart leaps at the thought of becoming his wife in a matter of minutes. I've waited for this moment since I was fourteen years old. No one has ever been as in love as we are, I'm certain of it. Standing beside him at the altar, I feel like a true princess. Tom is protective. He is an honorable man, who honors me as his wife, honors the country he serves, and honors the values, morals, and principles the military and the church stand for.

As our wedding concludes, he assures my parents he will always take care of me. Ten days later I left the home of my parents for the first time to live an ideal life in Europe. I was insanely thrilled and profoundly in love. Tom was everything I ever dreamed of having in a husband. Being with him was pure pleasure. I was young and vital, a nurse and the wife of a military man. My life could not have been more flawless!

Tom and I arrived at our first home in Holland late in the afternoon on a sunny day. It was a cottage with a thatched roof on a sod farm in the countryside. Pastures of green sod stretched all around us. Across one pasture a grove of trees lined a beautiful canal. It was magical at every turn.

We lived what seemed to be a true fairy tale in our little cottage. We walked through the peaceful trees hand-in-hand in the rain that sprinkled down at some point every day. We ate in restaurants housed in ancient buildings. We laughed hilariously with our friend, Mark, traveling to Paris, and Belgium, and Germany. The average, ordinary Minnesota girl in me was amazed that this was my life!

It was heaven.

We enjoyed our first newlywed weeks in Holland before I began to show symptoms of sickness. Tom came home from the base one afternoon with two bunches of pastel flowers in his arms, to find me vomiting into a plastic container in the second story bedroom of our little cottage. My head throbbed with a crushing, unspeakable force. It hurt to blink, to turn my head, to breathe. I hadn't been out of bed all day except to give insulin and to try to sip soda to maintain my blood sugar. I wasn't sure what the cause of the problem was.

The crazy-making pain and vomiting lasted for two more days before it subsided. Tom and I were both relieved. Two weeks later it started over again. I was diagnosed with migraine headaches. They were brutal and frequent. When they struck, I was completely incapacitated. The headaches dangerously compromised my health because vomiting and diabetes are poor partners. Diabetes itself destabilizes the delicate balance of electrolytes and the critical PH of the body. Vomiting doubles the threat to an already precarious state of health. After only a few weeks of being away, I was longing for the comfort and security of my mother, my home and my familiar doctors.

During these headache episodes, Tom tended to me in gentle ways. He was compassionate and concerned. He spent hours sympathetically stroking my head to offer some relief. His touch always soothed at least my emotional distress.

Then the sickness advanced beyond migraine headaches. My kidneys started to show damage from diabetes. The pressure on both of us was mounting rapidly. As I watched Tom walk toward me across the lawn, his image blurred. I was losing vision. To my horror, procedures I had done on my eyes just before our wedding weren't working. It made me sad, scared and even more lonesome for home.

Tom was stressed. I was afraid. I had no way to talk with my parents or to any of my friends at home in the States. We had only a radio and a tiny black and white TV set that came on after five in the evening to keep me company during Tom's twelve hour shifts. For weeks we didn't have a telephone. When we did get one, the international phone charges were excessive and calls to the states were rare and lasted less than ten minutes. I could no longer do the things I would normally do to occupy myself because of my failing vision.

I had no car with me on the sod farm because Tom needed it to get to the base every day. His shifts went from 11:30 in the morning when he'd leave until after midnight when he'd return. Life was a horribly isolating and solitary experience. I did my best each day to occupy my mind and subdue the boredom and loneliness, coupled with waning vision and mounting systemic health concerns. But my efforts were often futile. I managed to work for a short while on the base at the child care center.

One day Tom and I had a terrible fight. Tom grabbed me and shoved me up against the wall in the foyer, pinning me there and shouting in my face. I was shocked and terrified. I had never seen this aggression from him before. My rage hid my fear and I stormed indignantly from the house on foot.

I walked about two miles before sitting down behind a building and sobbing into my hands. I wanted my mother, my friends, to call someone, to go to a place that was familiar to me so I could feel safe from Tom and from the horrendous changes in my physical health that all came from out of the blue.

Tom eventually found me. Taking me into his strong, reassuring arms, he said, "Baby, it's okay. I am so sorry. I'm just scared. It's not your fault."

I remember looking into his eyes that were gentle and his body strong and loving. "I'm a rotten wife," I said to him.

"Don't talk crazy, you're not a rotten wife," he replied. "It's my job to figure things out, Shelli. You can rely on me. We can do this."

I felt comforted and strengthened with my head cradled lovingly against his heart and chest. I could feel his love pouring into me. I would need every drop of his strength and love to overcome what lay just around the corner.

We've been in Europe six months. I'm twenty-three years old, lying in an Army hospital bed in Frankfurt, Germany. My eyeballs feel like they've gone through a blender. The pain is searing into my skull and ears. Despite medication, the agony is unrelenting. Moaning, I try covering my eyes with the palms of my hands, but this doesn't help. Bulky gauze bandages cover my eyes. The tape securing them reaches across my temples, pulling on my hair, which makes me even more inconsolable. Trying to soothe myself, I rock slowly back and forth in the bed. Nothing helps. I'm thinking about the surgery I had the day before. A steel probe was cooled to sub-zero temperatures and touched dozens of times to the surface of my eyeballs, burning them and leaving them looking like raw, macerated meat. I'm alone in a large ward. I wish Tom would come, and have my mother with him.

I need to use the bathroom. I grope in the pitch darkness for the bell the nurses gave me to hold, one you might see at a reception desk with a sign saying, "Ring for service." I must have let go of the bell, but I don't remember doing so. Locating the bell in the tangle of sheets and blankets, I hit the top twice with my palm. After a few more furious rings the military nurse comes in. She helps me sit up and gain orientation. After some time, I stand. The world has disappeared. I have a hard time telling whether or not I'm standing upright. I stand in one place for a long time, breathing, trying to find myself in the empty void of nothingness that surrounds me. The pain is worse when I stand. I focus on the voice of the nurse telling me, "I'm right here." Staring into a black abyss, I reach for her voice, praying she keeps talking. As long as I can hear her I know I'm here, that something exists where I am and that I'm not floating alone in an empty universe.

My body feels disconnected from me. The nurse keeps both of her hands in mine so I have something to which I can anchor myself. I shuffle with infinitesimal slowness as the nurse walks backward, holding both of my outstretched hands in hers, down the hospital corridor to the group lavatory. I feel like an infant, incapable of even the most basic functions.

I stand zombie-like as the nurse backs me up into the stall. I feel as though I'm an animal being led dumbly into a trailer. My eyes are on fire, the pain so great I'm breathless. She takes one of my hands and places it on the wall of the stall. "Here is the toilet paper." She says.

"Where does it come out?" I ask.

She takes my hand and places it underneath the cold, industrial container. "Right under here. Can you feel it?"

"Yes, but I can't find the end." I reply as my hand blindly gropes and searches the roll of thin paper.

Finally, the nurse does it herself; pulling off the amount of toilet paper she's decided I will need. "Should I close the door?" she asks me.

"Yes, close the door and leave me alone for a bit." I say into the blackness, my bandaged eyes facing her.

"I'm afraid I can't do that. It's against regulations. We don't want you to be alone. I can close the door but I'll stay right out here and wait for you." She tells me.

"Fine, just stay there," I say with exasperation, as I use my hands to find the edge of the toilet seat and cautiously lower myself down. I pass gas and defecate. Humiliated and invaded, I weep silent tears.

Back in my bed I wail for the next thirty minutes. I want to disappear. I want to be home again, back to the dotted Swiss wallpaper in my little bedroom and grilled hamburgers and my wedding day that was just six months ago. I want to wake up and realize this is all a nightmare. I want to go to sleep long enough for it all to be normal again.

"Diabetes is a disease of the blood vessels." The microscopic blood vessels of my retina had become weakened and thinned by the corrosive effects of sugar surging through them. Eventually, they began to leak, spraying showers of blood like a soaker hose used on the lawn. These ruptures filled my vision with black streaks at first, and eventually there was so much blood I saw red pools in my vision. Despite many surgeries and procedures that were wretched to epic proportion, my retinas died.

When I first noticed changes in my vision, I was working in the emergency room. It was four months before my wedding. Reading the blood pressure machine became more and more difficult. Standing at one end of the department, the clock on the far wall was completely blurry. Some days I couldn't even read it. Driving to work, I could no longer read the street signs at the intersections. If the sun was shining on the traffic light, I couldn't tell which signal was on. I stretched my neck, thrusting my head over the steering wheel, squinting. "There! I can see it. It's not so bad." I knew I was dangerous and should not be driving, but that would be admitting the truth. If I said how bad it was, I'd have to let someone see how terrified I was. What's more, I'd have to let myself fully feel my panic.

I didn't want to feel the terror or admit the truth. I wanted to stay in my happy, sweet world of pretense, planning my wedding, dreaming of the life I would have being married to my first love, working as a nurse and living in Europe. I tasted wedding cakes and giggled through bridal showers with my best friends, all the while pretending I had not a care in the world. What a lie!

Despite my outward appearance, inside I knew I had to address the fact that my vision was decreasing and I knew why.

What frightens you so profoundly that you deny its existence and its impact on your life? Short of this, what is it in your story that you simply avoid thinking about, hoping it will go away? Denial is an excellent coping strategy, but it is ephemeral. Often we create the fallacy that if we don't think about the reality of our current situation or the facts of past events, they will dissolve. If only! What we avoid persists, and the residue shows up in mysterious ways. Sometimes the repression and denial take the form of physical illnesses, sometimes mental maladies.

It's frightening to face the truth about aspects of life that threaten our existence or way of living. Likewise, admitting we have a problem can jeopardize our self-identity. We spend more money than we make, but our pride and fear of appearing unsuccessful drive us to keep up our image, all the while credit cards and bills stack up. We are in a loveless marriage but the fear of being on our own, or being seen as a failure entices us to cover our illusionary life with lipstick or a new car. We believe difficult events that happened when we were children are long behind us and there's no need to consider them. *Besides,* we wonder, *what good could come from dredging up all of that old pain?* We can create all sorts of distraction that keeps denial riveted. But the truth always seeks exposure. The secret always wants to be liberated. The soul always yearns to live openly.

Before we can begin our healing, we have to admit the truth of our seemingly ruinous situation. If we deny that we are hurting or afraid, or that our lives are out of order, anger can fester into resentments and unexpressed grief can germinate into depression. If we consistently deny our negative experiences over an extended period of time, we can end up feeling lost or inauthentic. We eventually don't know what our truth is. We don't even know who we are or what we want. When we deny the truth of an injurious event or our truthful emotions of that event, we disconnect from the acceptance of both. Now neither the experience nor our emotional reaction to the experience feels real. When our emotions aren't real, and our experiences aren't real, we lose touch with who we truly are; we question whether or not we are real. This sets up a difficult conflict: If we're not real, we wonder, who are we? Deeper than that, do we even have souls? And, even more frightening, *If I look inside, will there be anything there?*

Admitting the truth of our situation is more than merely talking about our story, or talking about our distress. We have to feel it, and we have to express the feeling rather than just talk about it. There is a big difference between feeling sad or happy and expressing sadness or happiness. What do you feel in your body and where do you feel it when you express a particular emotion?

From an energetic perspective, every experience we've had--from the instant of our conception--remains in our energy system and it will remain there until it is released. Repressing or denying experiences, along with any emotions related to those experiences, requires a lot of our energy to hold them in place. Our energy bodies naturally want to move energy, not constrict it. The energy we use to depress our normal human emotions is the same energy we could be using to do other things, like caring for our children and our homes, enjoying leisure activities and most important, staying healthy!

Some of us are naturally emotional people. When this is true, the objective isn't to add to the emotional turbulence by encouraging more emotional expression. Rather, we need to be guided to find ways of calming the emotional flood. On the other hand, being able to express emotions can feel unnatural for some people. Learning to both feel and express emotions is part of one's healing journey. Contrary to outdated psychological theories, today we know that screaming and punching a pillow or beating the crap out of a tree with a bat isn't, necessarily, an indicator of healthy emotional release. Nor is it always required. The skillful practitioner will guide clients to find the appropriate balance of inner emotional experience with outward emotional demonstration.

Getting honest with the self and others takes time--time to realize we've been deceptive, time to figure out what the truth is, and time to work up the nerve to be honest. Honesty requires grit because truthfulness can make us vulnerable. If we want to heal the uncomfortable aspects of our stories and live an authentic, fulfilling life, skipping this step is not an option. Is it time to get honest? Is it time to take the dirt from beneath the carpet and let the truth clear the air?

As the reality of my failing vision set in, I saw Dr. Baumgartner and was referred to a retinologist. The first procedures I had were laser treatments. I sat upright in a chair, my eyes rolled to the back of my head, while a four-inch, thin, flexible needle was inserted just below my eyeball. The doctor pushed the entire needle into my eye socket until it was nearly in the middle of my skull behind my eyeball. The physician injected lidocaine, which was supposed to provide comfort. The needle made a squeaking sound as it skidded into my skin and slid behind my eye. It was far from being a picnic. The sound, the pain and the idea of a needle being thrust behind both of my beautiful, blue eyes made me queasy and want to faint. Holding my breath, I summoned up my warrior who could handle anything. I drove myself to every appointment alone. I was terrified every time. When my parents asked how it went I said, "It was fine." Then I went to work or studied for my nursing boards or fed the puppies in the kennel.

Now Tom and I were youthful, vibrant newlyweds living in The Netherlands. I believed the interventions I had before our wedding would be effective. But this wasn't the case. My vision started decreasing fairly rapidly. This small Air Force base had no hospital facility, only a small clinic. We traveled via train every month to Frankfurt, Germany, where I was treated at the 97th General Army hospital. It soon became evident that I would need better access to more sophisticated medical care. We received a humanitarian transfer from Holland to San Antonio, Texas where the Air Force medical center is located.

We were both deeply disappointed to leave our enchanted thatched roof cottage and our expected three-year tour of a charmed life in Europe to take up residence in the upper level of a 4-plex with white tile floors at the edge of a parched, dry Air Force base. Across the street was a dry field of thistles with railroad tracks running through it. The Texas sun scorched the land. Looking out at my new home through my blurred vision, I wept.

For over a year, my life was consumed with multiple operations in an attempt to save my eyesight. I went into each procedure clinging frantically to hope. One surgery lasted fourteen hours as a retinal surgeon did micro-surgery, peeling small, damaged cells off my retinas.

Thousands of laser beams were shot into my eyes during several procedures similar to the one I had before I was married. Other procedures were so painful the doctors used liquid cocaine to try to anesthetize my eyeballs. Glaucoma created unrelenting pain and pressure so great I was sure my eyeballs would explode in my head.

I refer to the fifteen months we lived in Texas as the decade of hell. Besides losing my eyesight, my kidneys were also failing because of damage caused by diabetes. My flawless life was shattered.

Each day was a perpetual measurement of what I could see or not see. I constantly picked up papers, cans, cards to see how well I could make out the writing. I'd look at them at ten in the morning, then again at noon, 1:30 in the afternoon and again twenty minutes later.

Alone in the apartment with nothing to distract my anxiety and worry, I stood at the patio door, looking out across the courtyard. Could I see the tree in the middle of the yard? How about the door on the house beside us? How clear was the door? Was it fuzzier than an hour ago? Eventually I could no longer see objects, only light and smatterings of color. The same game ensued. How much light could I see today? Can I still see the light from the dining room window? Can I see the light in the morning when the sun isn't coming through strongly, or only in the afternoon?

When Tom came home I'd study his face. How much of his eyes can I still see? Can I read his name tag? How close do I have to be to him to see any particular detail? Did the last procedure improve my vision as we all hoped it would? I strained with effort to see more, try harder. It was exhausting.

Mom flew from Minneapolis to San Antonio. While Tom went to

work, she drove me for an hour across unfamiliar highways to reach the Air Force hospital where I was being treated. We were there sometimes three days a week. Life was surgery after surgery, procedure after procedure, appointment after appointment. This was the sum total of my life at twenty-four years old after less than a year of marriage. It was dismal. I felt completely unprepared and incapable of handling everything that was happening. But what choice did I have? I'm a warrior; warriors do not back down.

In early July of 1986, I lay in another military hospital bed recovering from my current eye surgery. I had already lost all of my vision in my right eye. It was blind. The doctors were doing everything they could to save my left eye. My eye was blood red. The pain was searing and throbbing non-stop. The doctor came into my room.

"There's nothing more we can do. This is the last surgery. If this doesn't work, we have to face reality."

I was horrified. I wanted to stand up and slap my hand over his mouth and make the words stop coming out. I looked frantically at the blurred images of my mother and my husband, grasping for encouragement. My mother had been strong my entire life. No matter what I was going through physically, Mom was calm, reassuring, steady. If she was ever afraid, I never knew it. I looked at Mom there in the hospital room; I couldn't see the rivers of tears streaming down her beautiful face, but I listened to her weeping. Witnessing her reaction, I knew I was screwed.

I made a collect call to my father from the only phone for patient use, a pay phone in the family lounge. I sat in a wheelchair, my head hanging, a fraction of the woman I had been a year ago. "I have to have at least one eye." I wailed into the phone. "Please fix it for me," the little girl in me begged to make it all better.

"I wish I could, honey," he said. I heard his distress through the phone. There was nothing he could do.

Dejected and disillusioned, I hung up the phone. Sobbing, Tom pushed me back to my room where I found my Mom sitting alone, crying. Clearly, the world as I knew it had collapsed. I felt toppled, adrift. I believed I had no resources within me that reassured me I could manage all that was happening.

Weeks passed after the last procedure. Each day tedious and miserable with no reprieve from the violent vomiting, the kidney failure, the migraines and now ridiculously painful glaucoma. I continued with my obsessive, hourly assessments of what I was able to see, the words of the doctor echoing in my mind. Each day was worse, not better. I was totally blind in one eye now. What had remained in the good eye was fading each week, sometimes each day.

One day I sat in the doctor's office at one of multiple follow up appointments. The doctor examined the inside of my eye. He checked my visual acuity. As he finished the exam, the doctor slumped back in his chair, his hands limp in his splayed legs. He said, "I think the game is over."

An oppressive, suffocating weight instantly lifted from my body.

It had been far too much, for too long, with no good news. I was tired of the procedures that afforded no positive change. I was tired of the continual striving to see. I was weary of the effort required in keeping hope alive. I felt like I had been holding my breath for months and I could finally exhale. At least I knew now what I was going to deal with. I could move on and accept my fate, no matter how horrendous it was. I had a direction. In reality, I had no idea what it would actually be like to have all the light leave my world.

Nothing could prepare me for the isolating, dependent, terrifying darkness that would swallow me.

I flew home to Minnesota for a six-week visit soon after that appointment. No one said it outright, but everyone knew the reason for the trip was to see my family, friends and home for the last time. Coming back to my ordinary average surroundings gave me the emotional lift

I needed. I returned to the back steps of my childhood home, a place where I had spent hours upon hours in reflection while growing up, watching birds hop and the roses bloom. When I arrived I could make out the color and shape of the roses, although fuzzy. By the time I left, they had disappeared into dark grey shadows. The rejuvenation I felt quickly disappeared as well. In my mind I had wanted to go "back home," but I'd never be able to go home again. For me, home sweet home was snuffed out, overtaken by darkness. It would never be the same again. I would never be the same, either.

One night during the latter part of my visit I sought refuge in my old bedroom. The dotted Swiss wallpaper was gone, replaced with painted walls and a sofa bed. In the dark, I lay on my side as I wept silent, despondent tears of grief.

Dad came in and sat on the floor, leaning his back against the sofa bed.

"What am I going to do?" I asked him.

"You'll do just fine, Jack." Jack was the nickname he had given me some years earlier. His words made me cry harder. I had something to say to him, but my warrior was holding it back. Broken now by the weight of what I could no longer deny, I managed to choke out my words that were the cause of my real agony that night.

"I'm never going to be able to do what I planned. I won't be a nurse. I don't know what I'll do. I'm afraid I'm a disappointment to you now." It was true. In all my suffering with blindness, one of the things that frightened me the most was that I would not be successful in life. I believed my dad would see this as a failure and he would be disappointed. How would I ever earn his love now?

Dad turned to look at me, lightly running a single finger over the skin of my twenty-four year old arm. He said, "You have far surpassed any expectations I've ever had for you, Jack. You couldn't possibly disappoint me." Choking sobs fell from my chest. My heart felt a relief so intense it penetrated my belly. My body melted into relaxation I didn't remember feeling before. I had one less thing to anguish over; I met his expectations. I hadn't disappointed him. I wasn't a failure or a fraud.

By December of 1986, fifteen months after my enchanting wedding when I married my first love, I entered my new reality; a reality of absolute darkness, a blackness so all-pervading it felt solid. A reality that put me, "in here" while everyone and everything was "out there." It was a feeling of restriction and isolation that nearly drove me to insanity. I wanted out, but there was no "out" to get to.

I felt like the whole world had slipped into dark madness, too. Normal sounds like birds chirping outside the window became evil creatures come to take over my bedroom. I felt trapped and believed evil was going to overtake me. The impassable darkness pressed down on me. I was often filled with anxiety, wanting to punch through it and get to the other side. These crazy thoughts of evil and demons and feeling like I was a lunatic were completely foreign to me. I had been a grounded, sane person. I was not someone who conjured up incredible tales in my imagination. The idea that I was losing control of my mind along with my vision more than doubled my anxiety and fright. "What the hell is happening to me?" I asked myself often. One day, darkness took on physical form.

I'm lying on the sofa in the middle of the afternoon in our 2nd story apartment in San Antonio, wishing for sleep to come. The sleep will rescue me from the endless pain surging through my eyes. If I sleep, the time will pass. If time passes, Tom will come home from work and I won't be alone in what feels like a universe of emptiness. If I go to sleep, I can sleep long enough to change reality and all of this will vaporize. I will wake up and my "real" life will be back.

"Sleep, try to sleep," I coax myself. It's no use. The day drags on with insufferable monotony. Punching the audible clock on the table beside the sofa, with agony I realize it's been only ten minutes since I last punched it. My eyes are on fire, they throb with every heartbeat. I try turning on the TV. The sound of the game show coming toward me from the blackness makes me jittery. I turn it off.

Flopping back on the sofa, I hear the door open at the bottom of the tiled stairs that lead up to our apartment.

It's the middle of the day; no one should be here now. "Tom?" I ask into the darkness. No response. Frozen in terror, I strain to listen. Someone has broken in! I'm certain I heard the unmistakable sound of the door open and close. I listen with concentration, reaching to figure out what is happening in my home. I hear clip clopping coming up the tiled stairs. I'm catapulted into terror! I barely breathe, keeping as still as possible to try to figure out what the hell is climbing the stairs. The sound is unfamiliar. It isn't typical footsteps, but clip, clop, like some sort of animal, a goat maybe, slowly ascending the stairs.

I'm completely freaked out, and feel utterly panicked. What sort of beast got into our home? Is someone with it? My mind is racing. My heart is hammering in my chest. I feel sick to my stomach and wish I were able to stand up and run. But I can't. I'm paralyzed in fear. Besides, how will I run and to where?

The insistent clip clopping reaches the top of the stairs. Whatever it is, I can feel it in the room with me. It is less than sixteen feet away from me on the other side of the living room from where I lay.

I'm struck with immobility. I squeeze my already sightless eyes closed tightly. My chest barely moves as I try to breathe. Wild with fear, I play dead. Or pretend that it isn't here. *Ignore it,* I say in my hysterical mind. *This cannot possibly be happening.*

But it is real. The clip-clopping footsteps cross the room and head directly to me.

I feel helpless, naked, exposed. I feel as though all my strength has been sucked from me. I can feel this thing, whatever it is, coming closer. It has an unmistakable energy. My heart pounds, I'm hyper-aware of everything around me: the sag in the sofa, the sound of the air conditioner, the prickliness on my skin. I'm using every instinct and sense I have to figure out what it is that is now standing right beside me, hovering, as I lay like a pillar of stone.

It's so close now I can feel it. I don't know what in God's name it is, but it's mean, sinister, threatening. I can hear its heavy breathing. And feel its hot, muggy breath on my face. I can sense it looking directly at me. Its presence is ominous. I have no idea what to do, so I continue to deny its presence. If I don't acknowledge it, it isn't real. But it is real. I feel its menacing breath itch over my skin. I hear its labored, gruff breathing. I feel its massive presence at my side. I can tell it wants me. It came here purposely.

I lay for what seems like many minutes as the beast looms beside me, breathing. Waiting. A rush of fear whisks down my spine. I desperately want to scream, but I have no voice. I want to jump from the sofa and run like hell away from it, but my terror and blindness make it impossible. My anxiety soars. Desperate, my mind spins trying to figure out how to save myself from this entity, this beast or whatever it is. I know I can't overpower it with strength by choking it or fighting it. It's too massive.

Suddenly, I realize I have to admit it is here; it's real, I'm not imagining this. I know it will stay here forever, or worse, suck me up into its hot, clammy breath and carry me away, until I acknowledge it.

I turn to the beast, literally trembling and with fear I've never known, summon courage I didn't know I had. I shout, "I know you're here! I know what you are!" The very second I utter the words, a vision of an angel and a Christian cross appear in the blackness behind my eyes. It flashes in a millisecond, yet is intensely real. I'm filled with hope. Now I say to the beast, "You can't have me! I walk in the light of God." Instantly, in a split second, the beast is gone! Vanished. Evaporated into nothing. The room is normal. The sound of the heavy, hot breath is gone. The hostile, scary energy is gone. I hear nothing other than the sound of chirping birds and a barking dog outside.

In a frenzy of panic, I rush as fast as I can to the patio door leading to the deck. Throwing the door open, I thrust myself into the hot Texas sunlight. I stand listening to the sounds of normal reality. I feel the steaming heat of the Texas air and the deck boards burning my bare feet. I focus on the sound of the air conditioning units humming in a normal world. But in the darkness of my world, I search desperately, latching on to anything that will hold me here--here, I'm here. I'm real. This is real. I seek out a way to connect myself from inside the cave of darkness to the reality that exists on the other side of the black wall.

I don't remember how I found the courage to go back into the apartment that afternoon. Although the beast disappeared because of what I had done; I admitted it was there, and claimed my sovereignty. However, I still lived most days with the fear that it would return. Every day I continued to wrestle with the oppression that wanted to take over my life. This wasn't a battle anyone could fight for me, or even with me. I had to lay claim to my life, to my sanity.

I knew I had to get a grip on my mind and reclaim what defined me as "Shelli." I was losing myself and I knew it. Yet it seemed that everything that had previously defined me was gone. I wasn't a nurse. I wasn't physically healthy, in fact, I was critically ill and was worn out and beaten down. My independence was annihilated. I wasn't living a fairy tale wedded life in Europe. I was away from my family, friends, home, everything. I sat in a dark, noiseless, secluded, and lonely apartment every day while Tom worked. My only escape was the multiple trips to the hospital and doctor's office. I had nowhere to go and no one to be with. This was the truth of my situation. Nevertheless, I knew I couldn't wait for the conditions to change before I found the determination to keep moving forward. There was one thing I knew I had to keep: my spirit. If I lost that, I would truly be lost.

It would be many years and require a lot of healing before I understood the beast that came that day. The beast is representative of the insanity I felt as I lost my sight, the hopelessness I felt, and the utter vulnerability. The beast was illustrative of how blindness and illness stripped me of my identity. My life was being taken over by a kind of menacing force so great I knew it had the power to consume me... but only if I let it. It demonstrates the potential insanity that lives in all of us when faced with situations that are so outrageous we believe we won't survive.

Blindness, of course, is a monumental loss. Yet there are countless situations less terrifying that have the potential to create worry, threaten our stability and our hold on reality. Anything destructive that is relentless, that we are powerless to change, can drive us to madness. In the healing process, it becomes important to acknowledge if we are feeling as though all of normality has been obliterated and we stand teetering on the edge of insanity.

Short of feeling as though we're losing our connection with lucidity, any perpetual stressor or fear can circle ceaselessly in our minds. We go to bed but sleep eludes us. It becomes incumbent upon us to acknowledge the "beast" in the room or the recycling worries. When we do, the intensity of the emotions diminishes. We literally take the thoughts and feelings out of the small container of the mind and put them outside this looping track by honestly naming them. This is what I did when I spoke aloud telling the beast, "I know you're there and I know what you are." When we truthfully speak about our crazy-making worries and chilling experiences, a natural healing shift occurs. The withheld anxiety and fear is released and is "out there" rather than trapped inside our minds. Now we have space available for problem-solving and room for faith to develop. This useful healing technique promotes inner authority and power to replace hopelessness and victimhood.

The idea is that even though we feel unnerved, or anxious or even a bit crazy, there's more to us than our thoughts and emotions; there's more to us than our current state of affairs. We don't need to be a slave to our real fears or destabilizing worries. Even though our circumstances may be dire, we need to keep in mind that we always have things that cannot be taken from us: our spirit and freedom to choose. Part of any healing is to discover we have the capacity to overcome our distraught emotions, calamitous experiences and purposely choose our outlook. When we do, we are giving up our belief that we are victim to our conditions. If we believe life "happens to us" and we are powerless, we will experience life as an endless stream of misfortunes and bad luck. This is victim-consciousness. There is no possibility of healing in this belief system. We can decide to be miserable or to change our attitude. Whatever needs to be done, so long as we have some remaining control of our faculties, the choice is ours.

My greatest fear of blindness was not so much the lack of seeing, but the isolation that came with it and the dread of a life of limitation and insanity-inducing boredom. How I would function certainly entered my mind, but I was smart enough to know that I could learn to do tasks without vision. The greater fear was of having a worthless, unhappy and meaningless life because of the incredible restrictions that came along with blindness, especially thirty years ago.

Over time I made a conscious decision that my life was going to be whatever I made it. Although it appeared I didn't have choices, I did. I could choose to wallow in my misery every day, looking at only one side of the situation. Or I could choose to do the best with what I had. I decided that seeing was only one part of being alive. My warrior returned, fighting now for a just cause. I had a long life yet to live; I might as well be alive as it happened. I was going to do this, damn it. I would not permit darkness to eclipse my entire life! And thus, I began this portion of my heroine's journey.

The hero or heroine's journey has been described in mythology as willingness to face our greatest fears, our most sinister demons. Our healing process can often be this dramatic, although it doesn't have to be. Sometimes we are healing challenges that aren't life-threatening or life-altering, but those challenges are just as important to heal. In every case of healing there is an element of ominousness, of fighting with a foe that feels too big for us – and what is too big to us is relative to the individual. Some of us may be trying to overcome addiction, and others are challenged by driving on a freeway. In any case, we have to face the thing that would overtake or at the very least, minimize our life.

Each of us needs a purpose, even if it's just the purpose of the day. Ultimately, we all desire a life that has some sort of meaning, a reason to keep going forward and to get up each day. Within that purpose we find our joy, our passion and love, and our contribution and connection to the whole of creation. These critical aspects of life are unattainable when we are fettered, restrained by our fears, trapped within the unhealed parts of our story. Purpose doesn't imply something uncommon, noteworthy, or grandiose. True purpose is often subtle and unassuming. In fact, the most enduring purposes are those that are quiet, gentle offerings that are consistent and maintained over time.

The way to purpose, love, and passion is through self-esteem. Healthy self-esteem is cultivated by two means: by receiving positive reinforcement during childhood, or by healing the stories that heretofore have kept us believing we are small, undeserving, incapable, and unimportant.

As you begin to consider your own healing, you, like me, will likely find yourself groping blindly for where to begin. Any time we change, we move into the dark. We start in a place called 'here.' This place has light because we know what to expect, we know what to avoid, how to stay safe, and what the rules are. When we heal, we move from 'here' to a new place. The new place can feel as though we are lost in darkness, because it's unfamiliar. If we want to heal, we have to be willing to tolerate the unknown and the uncomfortable, face our fears, and become our own heroes.

Healing can be compared to walking down a dark, desolate alley in a bad neighborhood late at night. As we peer down the passage, everything in us screams to run, turn around, get out of this bad place! Beyond this frightening alley lies an oasis of everything we want in life. Sometimes we are aware of this oasis, but often we are not. We are mostly oblivious to the peace, the abundance, and the happiness available beyond the turmoil of our un-healed stories. When we enter the hero or heroine's journey of healing, we cannot imagine getting from where we stand at the mouth of the alley to the oasis beyond. In fact, we don't even know what we are aiming for.

In the beginning of our healing journey sometimes all we can see are the difficulties we'll have to face. We shrink back from the challenge, believing we don't have what it takes to face what lies between our captivity and our deliverance. A piece of us believes it isn't worth it. *I'm fine right here,* we try to convince ourselves. But then, the tension and pain of our discontentedness becomes too great. We decide we can make a run for it. We either barge ahead or take a few hesitant steps into the alley. Now we feel the heat and we freeze, just like I did when the beast stood breathing down my neck. Here we feel the duality of our longings; we know we need and want reprieve and liberation. We want passion, love, and joy, but we feel inadequate for the job at hand. As I discovered lying alone in the Texas apartment that steamy afternoon, I possessed enough of what was required to overcome my terror and continue my journey toward my healed self at the end of the alley.

As I steadied myself to get through each day in total isolation with no blindness rehabilitation skills, I realized I had to have a purpose, even if it was a pretend purpose that only occupied time. To keep my mind busy I counted pennies and nickels and put them into paper rolls. Then I'd empty the rolls out and start over. Dad sent me old comedy radio programs that had been recorded on cassette tapes. I played them over and over. Hearing the laughter grounded me. I took all of the clothes out of the dressers, unfolded them, folded them again and put them back in the drawers. Every day I did the same things multiple times. Yes, it was monotonous and boring, but I had to keep the beast at bay. So long as I had a purpose each day, even if it was something I fabricated, my incentive grew and I began to feel a bit more normal and a lot saner.

By September of 1986, I was attending vocational rehab in Minneapolis. Tom and I had moved home for the support we knew we would need. I ached for my freedom and independence. In the rehab program, I learned how to cook, do laundry, use a computer and read Braille. I learned how to make my home accessible through different things like brailing the microwave and putting marks on the stove and washing machine. I learned daily activities: putting on makeup, cleaning a bathroom, threading a needle, and using my hands as my eyes. As I learned each new skill, I felt hopeful that I could have a productive, happy life despite my circumstance. I came home at the end of each day with growing optimism born of my newest accomplishments. I was meeting other people who were blind who were further along in their skills than me. I found their stories and laughter inspiring. Tom was proud of me and we felt a mutual rejuvenation with hope for a meaningful life together.

I learned to use a white cane for mobility. Using it was supposed to give me independence and freedom, which it did to a limited extent, but mostly it reawakened my worst fears.

I'm on a training run with my orientation and mobility instructor from the rehab center. It's a hot summer afternoon. I've navigated the busy 4-lane intersections, tapping my white cane in front of me as I aim for the opposite side of the street, the traffic racing at my side. Using my newly acquired skills, I board a city bus heading for the downtown destination I've been assigned to reach today. I'm standing at the top of the bus steps, my white cane in one hand and the other on the step rail for balance and orientation. I gingerly take one step down when an elderly woman on the sidewalk waiting to get on grabs my hand that's holding my cane. "Here, honey, I'll help you," she says as she insistently yanks me down to the sidewalk. I'm indignant! I'm pissed at being manhandled and touched without permission. I wrench my hand free. "Don't touch me!" I shout at her, "And I'm not your honey!" My orientation is totally thrown off. I have to figure out which way I'm facing now. It's hard. I listen to the bus as it pulls away from the stop and use the sound to determine which way I want to travel. I'm annoyed, but determined to get through this damn mobility lesson. I walk toward the corner and swing my cane in front of me to locate the intersection. The wheelchair access makes my job more challenging; it's difficult to discern where the sidewalk ends and where the intersecting street begins. I rub the tip of my cane back and forth over the pavement, searching for the slight crack that lets me know I've reached the street. I finally decide I have it. I've calculated my route in my head before I left for my lesson. I know I want to turn left here to cross the street I'm walking along. As my cane sweeps the area in front of me to give me orientation, someone suddenly takes hold of my arm and starts walking me across the street. Furious, I wrestle with the idiot. "Let go of me. What are you doing?" The pedestrian says, "I thought I'd help you cross." "Well, I don't want to cross this God damn street, I want to cross the other street!" My instructor remains silent knowing I need to figure this out as though he's not there. I manage to regain my orientation yet again and continue on my route.

As I walk the sidewalk on this hot summer day, pedestrians speed by me. Bicycles zip along. With my white cane in hand, I stare straight ahead into the blackness, concentrating on my location on the busy downtown sidewalk. My cane clangs into objects on either side of me. Each time I have to stop and adjust my stride. I'm concentrating intensely, "Find the edge of this obstacle; don't worry about what it is. Find a clear path by sweeping your cane. Move ahead. Listen to the traffic; use it to guide you." I tap, tap, tap along. I bounce from one side of the sidewalk to the other, my cane whacking into unseen objects. It's painstakingly tedious, slow and awkward. I hate it. I feel like an imbecile, a poor victim plodding along like a blind earthworm. I keep walking, determined to make it happen. If I want independence, I have to succumb to this way of mobility for the rest of my life. My fury grows at the insane poking, tapping, sweeping with my cane to locate something against which to orient myself, or worse, a hazard to try to avoid. In my feeble poking, inching along between the multiple objects impeding me, another person stops, "Do you need help?" *See,* I think, *people pity me and think I'm a helpless victim.* I pass the person without acknowledging him. I hear women happily chatting as they briskly walk down the city street in their high heels. They are running errands during their lunch hour while I'm relegated to learning this maddening task. In a few more steps, I find myself hopelessly trapped between obstacles. I'm enraged! I raise my white cane above my head and hurl it into the middle of the traffic on the busy street. I scream at the top of my lungs, "I fucking hate this!"

My instructor retrieves the cane. He silently escorts me into an air-conditioned building next to us. I sit down on the floor, not caring who is there or what kind of business it is and wail into my hands. Mourning comes with a screaming cry from the depths of my soul. Is this really going to be my life, ping-ponging along a street riding public transportation? This isn't my life. I have more inside of me than what this limited life can provide. What's more, I have more to give.

Inside me lives a poet, an artist who sits in long periods of silence studying the minutiae of tree bark and shadows, the lace of fern and the movement of smoke. I'm a nurse who hasn't yet earned a single penny. I'm smart and know I have wisdom I want to share. I have creations inside calling to be birthed. I'm a leader, not someone who needs to be led by my hand. I have dreams, dreams of a normal life and dreams of my soul's longings: traveling to near and remote places, mission work, hiking mountain trails, watching football games, driving my car, and portaging canoes. Sitting here on the floor, I grieve with the intensity of what feels like a thousand burning suns for what I believe I will never have. I'm trapped in a sunless prison of a black eternity from which there is no escape. At this moment I'm sure that no one has ever felt this much devastation, anguish, or torment. I want someone to help me and once again, it seems heaven has closed its doors.

Blindness forced me to come to terms with my vulnerability. I had hidden my vulnerability all my life. I had created an elaborate image of fearlessness, power and fierceness. I refused to need help. Needing help meant weakness. Weakness was a set-up for betrayal and being hurt. Besides, admitting I had a need meant someone could take advantage of my need and refuse me, leaving me feeling abandoned. Here I was, unable to walk myself down a street without an elderly woman calling me "honey" and some unknown stranger taking pity on me. I was vulnerable. I couldn't pretend any more. The white cane shouted the truth of my fragility to the whole world.

The story of blindness doesn't have an ending. I can still fall to my knees for what I've lost and what I can't have. Practical things are to difficult: the loss of independence being sequestered in my home when I'd rather be browsing through a garden store or drawing a sailboat while sitting on a bench beside a lake. I want to be able to choose myself which shade of lipstick I think looks best. I miss the life I once had where there was sunlight and twilight and dawn, where there was movement and youth and aging. But what is most devastating is the loss of emotional experiences that come with living in a sightless world.

An unrelenting, torturous agony gnaws at my heart. It is a pain so unspeakable even my flesh cries in sorrow for the loss of never having seen my beloved second husand's face. I'm lost in the gallows of grief as I feel my interminable craving to have our eyes meet in the unspoken exchange of love. I long to study his facial expressions and the movements of his body that make him uniquely him. The sadness leaves me shattered. My world is often lonesome, absent of the acknowledgement of presence that comes with the exchange of a smile with someone I know as we pass one another in the hallway. I desperately desire to know the faces of my family today. I miss seeing the look of happiness or surprise or even grief. As Scott tells me about the look on my nephew's face after he makes a game-winning layup in an overtime basketball game, my jaw quivers and silent tears flow from my unseeing eyes as I listen to his excitement and realize I will never get to see what he saw.

I want to study the intricacies of a bumblebee as it works its magic through the throat of a flower in my garden. I want to see my garden--to watch it grow, bloom, and wither each year. I want to feel my smallness as I look out over an ocean. I want to watch the breath of a buffalo hang frosty in the air on a frozen day and be swept away in the silent beauty of it. I want to unexpectedly see a high school girlfriend and shriek with delight saying, "You look amazing." I miss the mystery of the night sky and the sunrise. I miss watching the soothing ripples of water on a pond, the beauty of falling snow, and the majesty found in gazing across a mountain range. I want to look at old photographs and remember. I want to watch people dancing in celebration. My breath and heart tighten with remorse as I yearn for the gaze of my dog looking at me with unconditional love as our eyes meet in wordless understanding of one another.

I want to notice someone looking at me so I know I'm not invisible.

Some losses are so great that the fist of pain will never loosen. Some wounds are so permanent, the best we can hope for is to maintain life between the moments when we once again return to the floor curled into a heap of mourning. The most difficult aspect of this profound grief is that it suddenly appears unbidden and unexpected. We are shopping for toiletries and a scent will hit us that unleashes a tidal wave. We are driving down the road and see an advertisement and in a flash, a memory is opened and the anguish that we thought had been dried up flows again. What is your loss that reappears without warning? Can you permit yourself to fall to your knees and let that be okay? Can you trust that once you've poured through the sorrow for the hundredth time, you will, in fact, be able to stand on solid legs again? Or do you push it all down, tightening your throat and clenching your jaw to keep it contained?

When in the throes of our misery, we can feel as though there is no possibility of light ever again. We can feel as though we are invisible in our mourning. Some loss and pain is singular and isolating. For me, losing my eyesight at twenty-four, while all of my friends were launching their adult lives with youthful eagerness and energy, left me behind and alone. I couldn't relate, although I desperately wanted to, to their reports of buying their first homes, the excitement of their first career jobs, or sharing the glory of their first pregnancies. Has your own story marginalized you from your peers? Have you ever felt secluded in your sadness while the rest of the world parades past, seemingly care-free?

If this is where you are in your story, it can be easy to blame, judge, and criticize others. Our jealousy and envy can take over. We want to rail at those who dare to have a happy life when ours is in the toilet. These are normal emotions at this stage of the healing process. We feel the torture of our situation and what's worse, our peers and what feels like the whole of society, aren't paying one damn bit of attention. If they were, our injured self believes their life would fall apart like ours.

We can become irrational, criticizing and blaming others for our situation. When we feel an injustice done to us--either at the hand of another or by unfortunate accidents, before we are healed we want to find someone to be accountable for our misfortune. This projected blame helps alleviate our suffering for a while, since the focus is directed outward rather than inward.

We know we're beginning to heal when we can stop blaming and judging others and instead become responsible for our emotions and the manifestations of our lives. When we have attained this level of healing, we have developed our consciousness to a point that gives us the ability to understand our story from a broader perspective. We begin to feel order in our lives rather than being recklessly tossed about.

It's important to know that each of us as individuals comprise the macrocosmic universal. It's not atypical for us to feel we are small and insignificant in the grand scheme of things. The truth is, each of us as individuals comprise the grand scheme. Our problem, our crisis, and our displacement affect the whole of humanity. And in so much as our personal fractures create universal fractures, so does our personal healing create universal healing. The degree to which we harbor judgments contributes to global opinions of right and wrong. The greater we can feel and know our individual sacredness, the more the world lives united. All healing begins with the self. If we cannot make peace within the self, we will not make peace with our spouses and brothers. And if we cannot make peace with them, how can we expect entire nations and cultures to make peace between them? So our individual healing becomes the salvation of the world.

THE HEALING

Blindness has provided me my most profound wounding and through that, my most profound gifts. Some holy stories of life arrive unexpectedly, leave an impression, and then move along. In these situations, time can be soothing. But as I said, the story of blindness never ends. I'm really no more healed, have not discovered more acceptance of blindness today than I had two years ago or twenty. When the physician told me I would be blind, I accepted my destiny. Just because I've accepted the truth of today's reality doesn't mean my hopes for a cure and restoration of my vision are latent. I'm not in mourning every moment, but I never was in perpetual suffrage. The grief comes intermittently, yet continuously, as life moves and changes without my observation of it all through my eyesight. Even today, I'll miss something new that opens the wound to a bleeding mess.

Sometimes I daydream about who I'd be if I hadn't lost my eyesight so young. When I'm in that state of melancholy, I believe that blindness has prohibited me from doing and becoming so many things I'd hoped for: taking my nursing to areas in need of mission help, expanding my art, volunteering in my community, living on acreage in the country, and attending more school. I once said to someone, "I'd be so much more if I could see." He said, "How much more could we take?"

What I have been able to do, through my healing process, is to integrate this devastation into my life and recognize the opportunities it's given me. Beneath the disappointment of unrequited dreams that vanished with the light, I've become many things I never would have considered, and in that is the healing. Few people are totally blind in the USA, especially people who become blind in their early twenties. The event gave me two choices: become a statistic and somber victim, or create new dreams. I chose the latter.

Through blindness I found courage I truly never knew was within me. When the beast arrived at my side, my bravery became greater than my terror. Alone, I realized it was I who had to overcome the demon that wanted to overtake me. In the face of an energy that appeared to be far bigger, much more powerful and stronger, I realized I had a weapon it did not: what I call Divine Sovereignty – dominion over my being and inner authority. I just had to summon the courage to call on it. Once I did, I recognized that I really wasn't alone, that the angelic beings who had always been with me had not abandoned me.

I had to face my fear in order to overcome what appeared to be too much for me. I could not be saved by denial or by staying frozen, hoping it would just go away. Denial did not rescue me, truth did. I'm not fearless, far from it. I learned that power does not come from pretending I'm not afraid; it comes from admitting my fear and moving ahead.

I don't need the courage or strength or knowledge of the world; all I need is the ability to take my next breath, or to take one, single step forward. I have learned that all I need is to simply speak the truth.

I had been a warrior all my life: denying my fear of inadequacy, of insecurity, hiding my fear with fierceness. As I was learning to use my white cane to walk down the city street, I was more afraid of looking like an incapable fool than I was of getting hit by a car. I found my real tears that day--the tears of a true warrior who's brave enough to fall down over and over and then stand up. The authentic warrior, the noble warrior, understands the power of vulnerability.

And finally, through blindness I learned that I'm much more than I thought I could be. Even though I wasn't able to do most of the things I had set my heart on doing, I'm still connected to a meaningful purpose that brings me satisfaction. I still worked as a nurse for twenty-five years after I lost my sight. Blindness taught me that adaptation is possible, and often the key to happiness.

I let go of how I thought I was going to live my life, of my aspirations for my work in this world. When I did, another gateway opened to possibilities for me to live, to provide worthwhile contributions to society. I discovered that if I would allow the healing, my greatest wounding could, indeed, be my greatest gift.

Had I not lost my sight, I'm unsure that I would have become a healer, a teacher or created a healing school. I might never have experienced the ecstasy of escorting people to their own healings.

I learned to give up demanding that the world see how much pain I was in and how I couldn't possibly experience joy in my condition. Before the healing, I wanted everybody to feel the same amount of hurt that I felt. And in truth, I wanted to punish people for being ecstatic as they gazed breathlessly at something that I, too, ached to see.

Being able to see with my eyes is only one part of life. I learned to be willing to allow the pleasure in other parts of life to fill and nurture me. When I did, life became fun again and I returned to being the happy, funny, irreverent and passionate person I knew myself to be.

I couldn't change the events of my life. Instead, I had to learn to change my perspective, and change myself.

Your spirit cannot be stolen unless you allow it. Let the warrior in you realize the power in vulnerability. Admit your fears to yourself, and to others. Weep when necessary. Laugh often. Embrace your pain. Know your greatest wounding and from that, rise up and adapt. Have the compassion to release others from needing to experience your pain for eternity. Let go of the idea that you can change others and past events.

Be brave. Be wise, and change yourself instead.

"Walking with a friend in the dark is better than walking alone in the light."
- Helen Keller

"New beginnings are often disguised as painful endings."
Lao Tzu

"Whatever it is you're scared of doing, do it."
Neil Gaiman

Chapter Four

BETWEEN HERE AND THERE

TEXAS, FEBRUARY 1987.

I'm kneeling on the bathroom **floor;** my face hovers over the toilet. I've been in the little bathroom over an hour already. I can't leave; my strength is gone, my muscles worthless rags. I collapse onto the pink bathroom rugs. My body is spent, and I allow the chilled air from the vent to comfort me. I'm limp and weary with fatigue. I've been vomiting like this for days, weeks, months. My bones poke through the wasted muscles of my scraggly frame and grind painfully on the tile. I lie on my back a while, my arm flung over my forehead, panting. After I begin to relax and can trust I'm done for at least the moment, I roll onto my side. I find the phone again and pick it up. Wearily I ask, "Are you still there?"

"I'm here," says the voice on the other end of the phone. I've never met the woman I'm talking to. She's been calling me for about four months now. Her name is Kathy Plumb. Kathy is in Minnesota. She's a volunteer peer counselor for people with complications of diabetes. At the moment, she is the only glimmer of hope I have that reassures me I will survive. I cling to her every word as though she were an oracle. The sound of her voice in my ear is medicine for my trampled, deflated spirit. It doesn't matter that I don't know her except through our phone calls. I'd talk with *anyone* who has survived a similar experience. "Please tell me I'm going to live through this," I say, a tattered pile of bones and flesh, my sense of self disappearing.

My world is melting from beneath my feet. I'm having visions of persecution from evil forces. The nerves in my stomach don't work properly. My kidneys are shot from diabetes. I need a kidney transplant. At times I'm afraid I'll die; and sometimes, I hope I do. My life is nearly unbearable hour-to-hour. I'm trying to manage diabetes, but the kidney failure and constant vomiting have made the unpredictable illness even more difficult to control. I'm going to be blind and everyone knows it. At twenty-four, life is a perpetual struggle, just a year into what I thought would be the romantic beginning of a perfect marriage.

I have to set the phone down and dry heave some more. My ribs and stomach muscles cry out in pain from the constant contraction. "Please don't hang up. Stay with me. Just stay on the phone with me." As long as I can hear Kathy's voice, I know there is a reality different from the one I'm in.

Kathy represents hope to me. She is also blind secondary to diabetes and had a successful kidney transplant some years earlier. As I listen to her speak, she sounds so normal; it's hard for me to believe I will ever live that way again. Inside, I feel odd, broken, and separate from how I observe others living around me.

For the fourteen months we lived in Texas, I was in the hospital more days than I was out. It was horrific. Tom and I were broke, sometimes getting food from a food shelf. It didn't matter that we were broke; I was often too sick to leave the house. Tom was resourceful, finding free things for us to do that I had energy to handle. One of our favorites was to visit a pet store and take the puppies into the playroom where I could sit holding them, letting their cheerful tongues and wagging tails brighten my spirits. It was extremely therapeutic. With this, and other simple events, Tom and I were determined and reinforced by the love we had for one another. His hand holding mine was better medicine than any pill I was given. He could change me just by being in the room. He was my solid rock, dedicated and always compassionate.

I overheard Tom talking to his mother some months after we had been re-assigned to the Air Force base in Texas. Tom's hometown had done a benefit breakfast in our honor to help pay medical costs. Tom said to his mother, "If anyone in town asks, tell them I love her way too much to ever leave her." I wept tears of relief as I lay in the adjacent room on our bed, a donated, stained mattress covered with a dense egg-crate foam to help minimize the pain in my body. I couldn't trust much in life at the moment, but I could trust Tom.

But as time passed Tom became more short-tempered. He was yelling at me for things beyond my control. He stood with his hands on his hips, his mouth in an angry line. I began to grow fearful of his unpredictable temper. My charming, honorable, and tender husband seemed to be vanishing. He was becoming prone to violent verbal outbursts. One day, the violence he held in his hands came out.

I was now mostly blind and terribly sick from kidney failure. I was isolated and afraid in the silent apartment all day. I had no means of communication with my family or friends at home in Minnesota. No electronic mail, cell phones, texting. We didn't have enough money to pay for long distance service on our home phone. We knew one other couple in Texas and both of them worked, so I was shut-in and without a single friend just as it had been in Holland. The hours of every day dragged by. I was bored, alone, afraid, and anxious, locked up inside the sterile apartment. Tom was my only connection. While he went to work and interacted with other people, I was at home vomiting, fending off the insanity in my mind and trying to function without eyesight with no rehab or emotional support. I felt like a terminally ill person in solitary confinement.

Tom comes home after work. I'm sitting on the sofa after another day of puking, pain, and stifling isolation. Something upsets Tom. I get angry that he is annoyed with me and I raise my voice to him. The next thing I know, a hand reaches from the darkness and strikes me across the face and head. I topple over on the sofa.

Completely shocked and utterly horrified, I begin to cry, which only makes Tom's fury grow. He shakes me violently. I'm speechless and distraught. I sit sobbing on the sofa. He goes to another room. I remain on the sofa with no place to go and no ability to get anywhere.

Later, he comes to apologize. "I snapped. I am so sorry. I don't know why I reacted that way," he says. I'm so sick and afraid I just want someone to hold me. My entire life is in ruins. I wish I could retrieve just one piece of what my life used to be. His embrace and genuine remorse is the one thing I have. I let myself be rocked in his arms that had always been my shelter. His protective and loving nature is back.

I was weak, sick and excessively fatigued most days. On the occasional good days, Tom and I did whatever we could to keep our optimism going. We played Trivial Pursuit, Tom reading my cards. Or we went to the mall and looked at things we couldn't afford to buy, but it was still better than the cold apartment. I hadn't learned to cook without my eyesight yet, but I helped as much as I could. The aggression that had come out of Tom earlier disappeared and I never saw it again, at least not in Texas.

During the years I spent away from home, in Holland and then in Texas, I often tried to comfort myself with memories of my life before

I lost my sight and my health collapsed. I thought often of the people, the places and the things I used to do. But I needed more than what memories gave me. I needed to be with people.

I craved contact with my family, my friends, and my average, ordinary life. As if the kidney failure and perpetual eye surgeries weren't killing me, I felt I'd also perish from loneliness and separation. The isolation became a continuous adversary that threatened my sanity and diminished my sense of support.

To ease my isolation, despite the gravity of my situation, my doctors, Tom, and I decided that it would be best for me to leave Texas and go home for an extended visit. We all knew this would be the last time I would ever see the faces of my parents, brother, friends and family because blindness was progressing rapidly. Soon after I arrived for my visit, an event occurred. It was so profound I carry the memory vividly to this day.

It's the middle of the night. I'm sleeping in the room that used to be my bedroom at my parent's home. I awake to an electrical sensation on one side of my body. I feel disoriented; my brain seems to have spaces in it where thoughts used to be. I sit up in the near total darkness of my limited vision. My legs won't support me. I fumble and stagger down the hall to the bathroom, using the walls to hold me up.

I sit naked on the toilet. My thoughts are jumbled, but I know something serious is happening. I'm anxious and panic-stricken. I try frantically to communicate with my parents, both of whom are now also crammed into the tiny bathroom. But my tongue and lips won't work. Desperately, I attempt to say, "911," but I can't get the words out. I hear myself and I know I'm not making sense. I'm anxious, but my internal world moves in slow motion. I search my muddy brain for how to communicate that I need an ambulance immediately.

As seconds slip by, my thoughts become more obscure and I lose more control over my body. Using my finger, I begin to deliberately trace the numbers, "911" on my leg while muttering the words. Finally, Mom and Dad understand and make the call. Mom dresses me as though I am an infant. My limbs are totally ineffectual, and I'm helped to their bedroom to wait.

I'm barely conscious in the Emergency Room. The things I'm aware of are very distant, as though I'm watching and not participating. I lose bowel control over and over again. A portion of me is horrified by this humiliation, and another piece of me is detached from the experience. I hear the voices of the doctors and nurses, but their voices are far, far away on the other side of an invisible barrier. Although I hear them shouting at me, I'm unable to answer their questions. One side of my body simultaneously feels as though it's not there and also like it was never a part of me. In the glimpses of orientation, I can't decide if this sensation is worrisome or not. And then I wonder why I can't determine what's threatening and what isn't. Eventually, all this becomes too much to bother with and I let go of the struggle to find the answer. It's a relief to let go.

I vacillate between obscure consciousness where I feel cold and afraid and at other times I glide effortlessly in a world of passivity where everything is quiet, calm, devoid of struggle. I enjoy this space that doesn't require presence or connection. I dance between this peaceful, effortless world and the world where I can hear doctors shouting and nurses calling my name, demanding that I respond. It's too loud, too difficult, too sharp and cold in the world of noise and voices. I am happier in the peaceful place of weightlessness and serenity. I want to leave the noise, but each time I do another voice pulls me back. Now they are pinching my fingers. The stimuli are intrusive and disrupt my peace. I want to go, but they won't let me. On the peaceful side I see light. I can float alongside delightful winged creatures that I cannot identify. I feel weightless and free. My body is strong and there is no effort. And more than that, I'm aware that the only emotion I feel is extreme happiness. I love it here! Then, a distant voice shouts and I'm annoyed at the effort

I have to use to listen and to comply with their intrusive demands to speak to them. I'm cold where the voices are. And it's dark and I feel terrific pain somewhere in my body, but I can't tell where. I hate it here.

After days of testing, hour-by-hour I stabilize and eventually return to present-time reality. I never was given a concise diagnosis or explanation of what happened that night. Doctors said there must have been some sort of stroke-like syndrome, but couldn't explain it. Amazingly, no cerebral damage was seen. I would have another such event before I would be set free from this bizarre period of my life.

When I returned to Texas after my visit with my family, I started dialysis three days a week. The experience was agonizing and gave me absolutely zero reprieve from the daily vomiting, excessive fatigue and misery that had become my life. In fact, life was worse. I believed the treatments would destroy me before they improved me.

I've finished dialysis for the day. It's a day like every dialysis day. Tom pushes me in a wheelchair to the car. He drove the hour journey here to drop me off in the morning and is back to pick me up. I'm like a rag doll as he nearly lifts my useless body into the car. At home, I can't walk up the stairs to get to our apartment. Tom carries me on his back. I lie on the sofa, wasted, demoralized, and miserable. Dinnertime comes. I'm uninterested. The diet I need to follow is tasteless. Besides, I don't have the energy to put a fork in my mouth. I move from the sofa to our bed and sleep for twelve hours. The next day the toxins start building up in my body, and the whole wretched cycle begins again.

I nearly live at the hospital. The emergency room visits and in-patient days stack up. I'm routinely having needles inserted into my lungs and the sack around my heart to drain off collected fluid that makes breathing and any exertion a chore. I'm vomiting hour-to-hour. Each day is a mind-bending test of endurance.

A little over a year ago I was a vital college graduate and eager bride who had inspired visions of her future bursting to begin. How did my life disintegrate to this? Diabetes.

The dialysis treatments never got easier; they never helped me to feel better. My life was simply a revolving door of riding to the hospital, taking the treatment, enduring the side effects and repeating it again in forty-eight hours. I was despondent and could feel myself slipping into a cavern of indifference. I needed salvation in the form of a kidney transplant.

In April of 1987 testing began to find me a possible living, related, kidney donor. In those days, only family members were allowed to donate kidneys. I had three chances: Dad, Mom, and my brother Scott. My parents both matched fifty percent, which was expected since I received ½ of my genes from each of them. Scott matched one hundred percent, a perfect match, like an identical twin. The news could not have been more fabulous for me. And for Scott, it was a decision that left him little room to say no.

Scott had an extreme aversion to invasive procedures. He wasn't afraid to give his organ to me; he was nervous about all the testing, needles, and procedures that involved objects being inserted into his body, things he would need to do just to learn if he could donate.

In late May 1987, Scott boarded a military airplane and flew from Minneapolis to San Antonio to begin a week of testing procedures. He was admitted to the military hospital on a Monday. I was having dialysis that day. After my dialysis run, Tom pushed me in a wheelchair to Scott's room.

With maximal effort, I hoisted myself up from my wheelchair, using my arms for the strength my legs no longer had. I was wearing shorts and a T-shirt. Scott stopped short before hugging me, "You're so skinny, honey. Look at your legs. You look like a bird. What's happening to you?"

"I need a kidney transplant, brother," I said with a wry smile.

Scott began the testing that included multiple vials of blood, tests to be sure he even had two kidneys, tests for possible future diabetes, tests to measure blood flow to his kidney, and tests to rule out any hidden illnesses he may have had. The tests were coming back great: all systems go. Until his HIV test came back positive.

In 1987 we barely knew what HIV was. At that time it was thought there was only one way to be infected with the virus. I looked at Scott and said, "What?" I could not have been more confused. Am I actually hearing that my brother who I've known for twenty-five years has been having sex with men and I didn't know it? *Can this story get any crazier?* The doctor said, "It's likely a lab error. All the tests came back positive today." Good grief!

The surgery was scheduled for June 4, my twenty-fifth birthday. What better day to be reborn! Surely, God was with me now.

The afternoon before the surgery I was getting what was supposed to be my last dialysis treatment when the transplant surgeon came to see me. "We have to put the surgery on hold," he said. I feel as though I've been kicked in the chest by an ox. How can this possibly be? We've planned, tested; we're all ready to go! Besides, I was barely alive. And that was the problem; I was too ill to survive the surgery. The doctors wanted to double my dialysis and hospitalize me for a few days to try to get me more stable for a better surgical outcome. I was gravely disappointed. Scott had already been in Texas nearly a week and now the surgery was being postponed. Mom was here anticipating the surgery. Dad was alone at home cutting hair, trying to maintain an income. We all just wanted the damn thing to happen already!

On the morning of June 11, 1987, I held the hands of my husband, brother, and mother. Mom kissed both of her children and said goodbye as we each were wheeled through the operating room doors. I can't imagine what she was feeling. Today kidney transplants are almost common-place, but in 1987 the idea of exchanging organs with living people was a new frontier. Here stood our mother with the heart of a lion as she smiled with reassuring confidence. I know a mother prays when she is powerless and can do nothing to help her children. I'm sure she talked to God often during the seven-hour surgery. To this day, her courage impresses me. We were so young: one of us dying and one of us holding the key that hopefully would give the one dying another chance at life.

After only five days following the surgery, I felt like a new person! My mother says the greatest sight she saw was my urine bag hanging on the bed beside me, full of clear, light urine that meant I had a working kidney. The second greatest sight she saw was Scott walking down the hallway on his own to visit me in my room just twenty-four hours after his operation.

I recovered very well and quite quickly. Soon I was putting on weight. I was back to being Shelli: funny, quick-witted, smiling, and energetic. I was off the kidney diet. The first thing I ate was a dill pickle and a Reuben sandwich. It was heaven!

Mom stayed with us for two weeks while Scott and I recovered together. We took daily walks around the base. We went off base to shop at a supermarket and bought 'normal' food. We ate fajitas and drank an occasional margarita. I had a life—a brilliant, real, happy life.

Yes, I was blind, but I was well! I could feel normality, though different than a year ago, returning. It was like stepping out of the cave I'd been wandering in for over a year, all the while wondering if I'd ever find my way out.

Tom and I wanted to get back to Minneapolis as soon as possible. It would require having to separate from the Air Force. Our choice meant we would have no medical insurance, no jobs, no place to live. The doctors tried to dissuade us. But we longed for home and the familiarity and support it would provide, as well as the chance for me to get quality vocational rehabilitation and to do something useful with my new life. Tom applied for a humanitarian discharge. His application was granted.

My new kidney has worked perfectly for the past two months.

Tom, his brother and I are in our now vacant apartment doing the final cleaning before leaving Texas. The movers have taken all of our belongings except for the suitcases we packed. Tomorrow morning Tom will see the base commander and sign his paperwork, discharging him, and me, from the Air Force. After that, we will make the twenty-four-hour drive home to Minneapolis. As I scurry on my hands and knees, cleaning the baseboards, I think of the city lakes, the clear, blue water, my favorite pizza place, my family, my dog, and my life-long friends, LaRae, Jade, and Cherie.

As the afternoon fades and we are finishing our work, I start feeling nauseated. I sit on the cold tile floor, my hands over my kidney in my tummy. I feel a slight discomfort. The pain and nausea are short-lived. After lying flat on the floor for some minutes, the symptoms pass. We all decide I likely strained something as I cleaned. We leave the apartment I hated since the day I saw it. *Good riddance,* I think as we close the door behind us. In just one day I will be sleeping in Minnesota again! The three of us get something to eat and Tom and his brother drink a beer before heading to the military hotel where we will spend the night.

It's midnight. My abdomen is distended and throbs in pain. I'm vomiting. Tom's brother kneels beside my bed, his hand on my waist, "You're going to be okay, Shelli," he says. Tom calls the surgeon on-call. He instructs us to get to the emergency room immediately. We all wonder if we should call an ambulance, but decide we can get to the hospital sooner if we just leave now and drive.

I'm in the emergency room yet again, Tom standing at the side of the bed. Distraught, I writhe in pain. A part of me wants to get up, walk out and pretend this is not happening. A part of me wants to move ahead two days and magically carry me to Minnesota where none of this will be real. I so wish that wishing could create reality.

Tests reveal that I have an "incarcerated hernia." A loop of my intestine is poking through my abdominal wall and is being strangulated. My new kidney is encapsulated by a large amount of blood so dense that doctors can't feel my kidney beneath it. The medical team can't tell where the blood is coming from. Something has gone terribly wrong inside me. I need emergency surgery to reduce the hernia, drain the blood, determine if the kidney is injured, and further, if my bowel is permanently damaged. If it is, I will come out of surgery with a colostomy.

I cannot believe this is happening. *Seriously? I was just re-born eight weeks ago! I was fine two days ago. We are leaving to go home tomorrow morning. Home. I want to go home.*

This is simply another nightmare I'm in. How much more can I possibly take? The torturous past eighteen months are scarcely behind me. I've only been standing for sixty days. How could I be face-down in the dirt so soon?

I franticly search for God, the God I'm not even sure is on my side. Nevertheless, I tell Him, *I'm holding on by my fingernails. Save me.* I wait. I listen to my breath. Then I distinctly hear, *Let go.* My willful self rails against this insanity. *Let go? I don't need to let go. I need to hold tighter!* In time, I realize it's my fear I need to let go of. This means I have to trust. Inexplicably, I am able to do just that.

Tom stands beside me as I lay waiting to be pushed into the operating room. He is going to see the base commander to sign himself out of the Air Force. Once he does, from that signature forward, we are on our own. We will have no medical insurance, no jobs, nowhere to live other than the fold-up sofa in the tiny den of my parents' home. Neither of us knows what is going to happen in surgery or what I will need afterward. We have no idea if my kidney is working. We don't know if I'll come out with a colostomy. *Let go,* I hear again.

"What are you going to do?" I ask Tom as I lay on the gurney, the drugs starting to work to relieve the pressure in my abdomen. Minutes go by in silence. I feel him considering his options. I think, *Let go.* "Screw it," he finally says, "I'm just going to do it." Tom kisses me goodbye and strides down the hall. The sound of his fading footsteps are resolute. I'm pushed through the operating room doors where I will be put to sleep while surgeons discover whether or not my kidney is still functional and if I will need a portion of my intestine cut away.

Meanwhile, my parents wait by the phone in Minnesota. Tom and I are on our own. We're twenty-five and twenty-seven years old. If we both weren't mature, independent and tenacious, we could have easily collapsed. We could have easily fallen into our insecurity and fear and stayed in the safety the military provided, and, I believe our spirits would have dried up in the Texas sun.

People are born with intrinsic character traits, and other qualities are developed through early conditioning. My parent's method of fostering independence may not have been ideal, but I did grow up and learned to make important decisions without their continual oversight. While I often struggled early in my life, taking on tasks that felt, and were, too big for my child-sized thought process, I also gained important skills and qualities that served me later in life. As you look back on your formative years, what important characteristic or skill did you acquire despite not having perfect parents? Can you see how what you perhaps didn't get from Mom, Dad or whoever raised you, paradoxically taught you life-skills that have sustained you? A natural healing moment occurs when we are able to recognize that our experiences of life have not been wholly bad nor useless. When we authentically reach this degree of healing, we know that we are moving out of the story as a means of self-identification. We are becoming more fully who we truly are.

Gratefully, I came out of surgery just fine. My bowel started working as soon as it was released. The blood that had been covering the kidney was from my abdominal wall where it had torn open, allowing the intestine to bulge through. There was nothing wrong with my new kidney! We celebrated our blessing and moved back to Minnesota, but the story of my kidney transplant wasn't over.

Despite the fact that I had a perfectly matched kidney, I had three rejection episodes in the first year after transplant. Treating rejection is a difficult endeavor, especially in 1987. Many of the medications used to interrupt the rejection were experimental. Some had even been banned, but were being used anyway. I would recover from one rejection episode and within eight to twelve weeks, my kidney would reject again. During my first rejection treatment, I had an out-of-body experience that taught me something about who I am beyond my physical body.

I'm lying in an intensive care unit. I've received three different medications to try to reverse the rejection and save my kidney; one of them is experimental. It's early morning, maybe 6 A.M. I have a bell on my bed to call the nurses.

Without warning or any sign of distress, I feel myself leave my physical body and drift upward. I find myself suspended like a cloud at the ceiling, my arms and legs dangling like a jellyfish. I observe myself at the ceiling as though I am a third-party spectator located randomly in the room. Instantaneously, all of my conscious awareness, that which is having the experience of being "me," is present only at the ceiling. My ceiling-self observes the body in the bed dispassionately. I know I'm looking at my body in the bed, but I'm not connected to why I'm "up here" while also seeing me "down there." All of me is at the ceiling observing what is happening to my body as though I'm a spectator of my own life.

As time goes on, my ceiling-self notices my bed-self is shrinking. My ceiling-self finds this fascinating for a while. Then, with sudden shock, my ceiling-self realizes that the "me" who's in the bed is so small, that if I get any smaller I will evaporate and be gone. In a millisecond of time, my ceiling-self switches from dispassion to abject terror, suddenly realizing that the person who is in the bed is also herself. At the ceiling I have a moment of epiphany: "I'm leaving my body and if I don't go back into it, I will not exist." In the next non-measurable unit of human time,

I decide I don't want to leave my physical body behind while I head for another dimension, and my ceiling-self unites with my bed-self.

I was viscerally and visually aware of all that happened during this experience. Once back in my body, everything seems to happen at once: I re-enter my body, and alarms begin to ring around me. A flurry of nurses rush to me administering IV medications. I had remained fully oriented while I was out of my body, but when I returned to it, my coherency faded. Once back in my body I drift in and out of awareness and often have no comprehension of what is happening. In reflection, I found it fascinating that my out-of-body experience happened in advance of the critical care alarms sounding. In other words, my consciousness knew what was going to occur before it actually happened.

My perfectly-matched kidney from Scott survived this rejection episode, but within a matter of weeks I was back in full rejection again. Saved from this second episode of rejection, ssome weeks later my kidney function rapidly declines and, as ludicrous as it seems, I'm in rejection yet again. The third go-around hit me hard emotionally. *Can I be granted a stinking break? I just want my already limited life back.* I began to wonder again, *Where has God disappeared to now?* I felt sad and plain worn-out. It had been three consistent years of sickness and major life challenges.

Doctors gave me a poor prognosis. I was told it was unlikely I'd keep my kidney. It seemed that with three rejection episodes all within months of each other, and despite powerful medications, my body was refusing to accept the foreign part. I couldn't just lie in the hospital bed, waiting and hoping my body would change its mind and let my new kidney become a part of me. Talking with a friend, positive imagery was suggested. It was 1988 and I didn't know much about what was then called alternative modalities. But I needed to do something that helped me to feel I was a part of the recovery process. It wasn't in my nature to sit at the side and hope that doctors, medicine, or someone else would handle everything for me. When I feel as though I can do something to help myself, even if it's a small thing, I feel empowered rather than victimized. I began to use positive imagery. The next day my kidney function began to show its first signs of improvement. From then on my kidney rested quietly in the home of my body.

Scott's kidney served me well for twenty-one years, an excellent record especially after three rejection episodes and the continuing damage of diabetes to this new kidney. Scott's gracious gift saved me from sitting on a waiting list and continuing to endure the ghastly experience I had on dialysis.

Because of Scott and his kidney, I lived abundantly through my twenty's, thirty's and into my latter forty's. I was able to work as a nurse, return to school, become an aunt. I celebrated twenty-one more birthdays, two more decades of holidays and remained present for my family and friends to love. In turn, I was able to love the important people in my life and to contribute to their life experiences. As I reflect, it's a humbling feeling to know that without Scott and the miracle of medicine, my life would have ended by the time I was twenty-five. I am eternally grateful, brother. Some years later I would go through yet another amazing healing experience. During this time I remembered Scott's gift and wrote to him, " I'd thank you from the bottom of my heart, but for you, my heart has no bottom." I don't recall the author of that quote.

I found renewed spirit after my first kidney transplant. We were discharged out of the service and returned home to Minnesota. The family support and familiar surroundings all helped me to feel confident and took the full burden of my special needs and health off Tom's shoulders. My entire family praised Tom for all he was doing for me and his dedication to me. To my family, Tom wore the wings of an angel. Everyone could see that Tom loved me in a profound way. Although I was only twenty-five and totally blind, I was smart and resolute to make something of my life. Tom encouraged me every step of the way.

We bought our first home and we set about making a life for ourselves. I attended rehab and gained skills at living in a world absent of light. I used my white cane to take the city bus to appointments. I walked independently to the corner dairy store and enjoyed working in our home, making meals, doing the cleaning and laundry. I felt like a human being again, and felt like the wife I wanted to be for Tom.

I decided that using a guide dog was a better fit for me than the white cane. I came home with Mel, a happy Golden Retriever after spending four weeks in California at Guide Dogs for the Blind training with him. Mel and I walked jauntily down the urban sidewalk to our house. Tom stood watching me. As Mel and I glided up to him and stopped, a wide smile spread across my face. Tom embraced me in a hug of sheer delight. "I don't want to ever see you with a cane in your hand again. You are beautiful," he proudly said.

I was determined to use my nursing education and be a productive part of society. I won a battle with the Minnesota State Board of Nursing who didn't think people who are blind ought to hold a nursing license. "I lost my sight, not my mind," I said to the Board. I became the first blind nurse registered in the state of Minnesota. I created my nursing position doing education in the cardiac unit in 1989, selling the idea and proving myself to the hospital.

I went to work every day. I planted flowers, learned to crochet and do other activities with my hands. We finally had money and did things normal people did. We took vacations to California and Idaho, hiking deep mountain trails, fly fishing together and camping alongside chilly, hidden mountain streams. Our life was finally blossoming into the experience we had always wanted it to be. We had survived the horrors of all that happened in Texas. I believed if we could survive all that happened there, we could endure anything.

Yet despite the happiness and successes, Tom's temper seemed to be unleashed at moments when I didn't expect it. His tender compassion was evident most days, but some days he was a fiercely snorting bull, suddenly raging over trivial incidents. It was as though his temper didn't have a middle ground. Many times I wasn't timid in my response. I was offended by his hostile, accusatory remarks and the frequent times he snapped at me for things I had no control over, like bumping him from behind when we were walking into my parents' house to visit. And at other times I became passive, trying to let the anger in him dispel with less incident.

His physical assaults returned as well. Sometimes his abuse was limited to pinning me against a wall, and other times he hit my face and head or pushed me. Sometimes he'd violently squeeze my arms and shake me. It became apparent to me that alcohol intensified his wrath.

Tom arrives home late one night after drinking. I am asleep in bed, but I wake up hearing him stumbling in the house. I can feel his agitation before he enters our bedroom. I know to be quiet. I don't want to upset him or say anything that will somehow set him off.

I lay silently as he gets into bed beside me. He shoves me, trying to start a conflict. I get out of bed and walk passively to the living room. Tom follows me and towers over me as I lay on the sofa. "What the hell are you doing out here?" he roars at me. I reply, "I'm fine. I'm just letting you be alone so you can sleep."

"Get back in the bedroom," he screams at the top of his lungs. I'm shaking with alarm. Although I have known Tom to be fierce and hostile, I have never seen him this aggressive. It's clear to me that he is totally out of control.

I stand up to go back to the bedroom. Tom pushes me down. I fall onto the floor and Tom begins kicking me. I'm lying on my side crying. I curl myself into the fetal position, trying to protect myself and get as small as possible. I'm afraid he is going to injure my kidney, which is sitting at the front of my body just beside my bellybutton. Standing over me, Tom puts his foot on the side of my face. He sneers in a maniacal voice, "You've ruined my life and you're going to pay."

I'm paralyzed with fear. He has my head pinned to the floor under his two-hundred pounds and is now starting to press his full body weight on my skull. I scream, "Tom, stop!" He moves his foot from my head and face to my throat. "You're going to pay right now," he says in a voice I don't recognize. I'm certain he's going to break my neck.

I'm rigid in terror. *Resist nothing,* I think, *Stay perfectly still.* Besides, what other option do I have? I use every ounce of courage I have to freeze my body and to diminish my sobs of terror as he steps on my throat. I whimper and let silent tears escape my eyes.

I don't know, or at least I don't remember, what tamed Tom's murderous rage that night. The next day I was so despondent I could barely function at work. I told no one, except one girlfriend I knew I could trust. I swore her to secrecy. I was humiliated and ashamed. *How could my glorious husband, the one who proclaimed his dedication and promised to care for me and protect me and honor me be battering me and telling me I had ruined his life? And, worse, was it true?*

Tom came home from work the next day equally humiliated. We both cried and he asked me to forgive him. He gave me believable explanations for his outrageous attack, saying he was stupidly drunk and he was foolish for allowing himself to get so out of control. He sounded so sincere, so remorseful. He hugged me as I cried and once again I allowed myself to be comforted, though my trust was eroding.

He assured me it would never happen again. Caught up in my denial and wishing to focus on my love for him, I believed him. I didn't want to face what I knew was true; Tom was abusive and violent.

Tom's rage and physical indiscretions didn't stop. His physical abuse wasn't constant, but it was unpredictable and always intimidating. His impatience grew, but he was also very attentive, tender, and caring.

It was confusing. Because I never had a broken bone or a black eye, I convinced myself his violence wasn't really all that bad. Love and denial does bizarre things to a person's mind. I resorted to the useful and untruthful coping strategy of denial. It worked, for a while.

THE HEALING

Before kidney failure, I didn't realize I could be as sick as I was and survive. The fortitude and wisdom of the physical body impressed me and taught me what a miraculous creation it is. I learned to honor it and all that it does, despite the lack of perfect conditions.

My spirit was equally torn during this extreme illness. Until this time I had enjoyed the close proximity of my family, my friends, and familiar doctors who had known me for years. I hadn't realized how much I relied on them, and needed them to be near when I was weak, or lonely, or overwhelmed.

The experience of being so far removed from my community in my most desperate time illuminated for me the irreplaceable importance of community, of belonging to a group, and how much that community provides its members. As a young woman in my early twenty's, I believed that independence, autonomy, and self-reliance were the important qualities needed to feel strong in the world, and what I thought others wanted me to be as well. I hadn't yet experienced emotional devastation and the need for community until I found myself without a community. The illness I felt in my body was challenging, to be sure. But the emotional discomfort I felt in the absence of those who loved me was often times a greater torture. The hours of emptiness, and oftentimes utter silence coupled with blindness, left me feeling hopeless and depressed. I learned that I could not heal without the presence of other human beings who cared for me, who loved me, and who I could care for and love in return. I longed for community to cry with, laugh with, and to share their own stories with me.

As I experienced myself outside my physical body while in the emergency department and in the ICU, I encountered a tangible truth that changed my perception of what it means to be me. I am not limited to the physical dimension. Beyond my effort to stay here, live, hold on, I found another dimension of existence that was often more vibrant and inviting than the material reality. I'm grateful for this early experience; later in life I would come to remember it and lean on it for reassurance.

As I became the recipient of the selflessness, the compassion of others, I understood the emotion of gratitude in a way that defies words. Kathy, the volunteer peer counselor, spent hours on the phone with me, a person she only knew as a voice on the phone for the first two years of our relationship. Through her, I learned that I could ask for help, even from a stranger, and have my call answered.

Scott and I had a close relationship, but I frequently believed our relationship was not balanced; it was as if I had more authority and power. When we were young, and through high school, learning and charisma came easy to me. I had sometimes seen Scott as being less capable. I thought of him as somehow weaker, more vulnerable, needing more help than I and I believed it was my duty to stand behind him, giving him the strength that came so easily to me. My perspective of him was transformed when he offered me his kidney. I witnessed his courage despite his tremendous fear.

When I received his kidney that was an identical match to mine, I felt a piece of me was returned. After some years, I began to realize that I had always felt a connection to Scott that was indeed, like an identical twin, rather than siblings born thirteen months apart. The bond of this connection is part of what drove me to believe I had to act as his "strong half." I felt whatever distress he felt. I was upset if he was unhappy or struggling. After his kidney came to be mine, I felt the union between us change. We became equal partners, mirror images in our lives. I needed him to support me in ways I had never seen or at least never admitted. I needed him beyond the gift of his kidney. Today I feel a bond with Scott that goes far beyond blood. I experience our souls as being bonded.

I came to realize that my perception of events and of people isn't always accurate. I was humbled to make this realization. After all, I thought my interpretations were the right ones, the only ones. As I recalled the out-of-body experience and the time spent in the reality of serenity without the loud voices and pain of the emergency room, I recognized that all events truly are relative. If I could be an animated version of myself at the ceiling, having an experience totally different than the experience I was concurrently having in the bed, it must surely be possible for two separate and distinct individuals to perceive things vastly differently. I had begun to learn that I was not the only observer and I surely could not know the depths of people's characters and strengths simply by my assessment of them.

Humility is a valuable quality. Humility has allowed me to receive. I'm still learning how to perfect it.

As we heal we are able to witness ourselves and others with refined clarity. This clarity allows us to see things about ourselves that we couldn't see before. This part of our psyche is known as, "the shadow." In chapter one I wrote about how I discovered a shadow aspect in me that tied fun to food. It was a remnant of how I had experienced my life with diabetes that was still alive within my psyche. The healing that happens when we become aware of shadow beliefs or thoughts may be even more important than mending the obvious injuries we've experienced. Self-inventory is painstakingly difficult and exceptionally emancipating. "Shadow" refers to those aspects of us that we don't know exist. They may be unsavory or undesirable qualities or beliefs, but they include unseen talents and gifts as well.

The inner work of self-inventory is like sitting in a dimly lit room.

As we look around, things don't appear all that out of order, but we can see some clutter we'd like to get rid of. We begin the healing process by adding light to the room with new awareness and insights. Now we can see the room more clearly and we're shocked! Our illuminations reveal that the room is filled with junk we've tossed in here for years, because we didn't know what to do with it or we were afraid of it. And we've also put our treasures in here too, because we didn't know how to accept or use them, either.

Personal healing is a choice. I continue to choose to do the work of self-inventory because it's important for me that I have every room of my internal home open and available. I want to keep the junk cleared so my golden qualities are easily accessible and readily seen. I want to be transparent about my human imperfections too, so that I'm a real person and seen as one.

Are you more comfortable sitting in the dimly lit room instead of doing self-inventory to reveal your shadow? What is the old junk you've shoved into the little room that is best to let go? You have a treasure trove of valuable qualities waiting to be revealed!

Your body is stronger than your mind believes, your mind is more powerful than you imagine, and your spirit is more invincible than you know.

"One of the greatest discoveries a man makes, one of his great surprises, is to find he can do what he was afraid he couldn't do."

Henry Ford

"What does not kill me makes me stronger."

Johann Wolfgang von Goethe

"I love those who can smile in trouble, who can gather strength from distress, and who can grow brave in reflection."

Leonardo da Vinci

Chapter Five

SHATTERED

ONE DAY, TOM LEFT OUR HOUSE IN A RAGE AND NEVER RETURNED. I was stunned and shattered. He refused to tell me where he was staying, why he left, or what his plans were. I suspected he was having an affair. He vehemently denied it. "The last thing I want is any more trouble. I'm just confused and I need time to think. Everything will be okay."

After six weeks of separation, Tom called and asked to have dinner with me at a restaurant. Waiting in my prettiest dress with my guide dog Mel at my side, I was terrified about what he might have to say. Oddly, I felt like I was about to hear a judge lay down my sentence, but I still didn't understand my crime.

We made some small talk and ordered dinner. I was beginning to feel more relaxed. Tom seemed relaxed and said a few things that made me smile and even laugh. In time, he looked directly at me and said, "I think we should live separately."

Hot burning rose in my stomach. Confused, I said, "Isn't that what we're doing now?""No," he said. "I mean separate checkbooks and bank accounts, things like that."

"Tom, what are you talking about, really?" I asked.

He finally said it. "I think we should get divorced."

I felt the blood drain from my face and my stomach turned. I needed things to slow down. Just weeks ago we were planning a romantic trip to the North Shore of Lake Superior to ski, huddle down in front of the roaring fire, drink wine and enjoy long mornings. The week before he left, Tom had given me an audio Valentine card he recorded in his own voice saying, "Be my Valentine because I love you very, very much, sweetie" and yet he now wanted a divorce?

After this meeting we decided to try counseling, which helped more than either of us anticipated. We were talking about real issues that had never been discussed. Although he didn't move back into the house, we saw each other. We "dated," going to dinner and attending events. Tom said he was feeling optimistic that we were going to work out our issues. We talked about new long-range plans. I learned about things that had bothered Tom that he'd never told me. We were getting along better than we had in several years. After being separated for a little over three months, we arranged to have dinner in our home. I was euphoric!

I anticipated a sensitive reunion back in our home. I set a lovely table on our screened porch, set out the wine glasses, lit candles, and put on a new sundress and Tom's favorite perfume.

Tom came through the door and appeared agitated. Before we even poured a glass of wine, he said, "I'm going to be a father."

My legs turned to liquid. Staggering, I sagged into a chair. I felt the stab of a knife in my heart that traveled to my belly. Something split open inside me that felt permanent. I sat frozen, voiceless, in complete disbelief and horror. He left thirty minutes later.

I felt him turn his back on me with insensitive, careless disregard.

It seemed he couldn't get away from me fast enough. The sound of the door closing behind him rattled my bones.

I threw the steaks away and poured the wine down my throat, uncertain of my next moment. I didn't even know who to call.

The mourning made me numb. The betrayal made me sick. I felt as though a piece of me was viciously torn from my heart, my soul, and went through the front door with him. Nothing I'd gone through, blindness, kidney failure, organ rejections--had been this defeating. I hurt emotionally, mentally, physically, and spiritually. Seeking reprieve from the ceaseless torment, I turned to the solace of wine. I called every friend over and over again. For weeks it was the only thing I could talk about. Each phone call reviewed the same stories, the same words and emotions. I refused to share the news with anyone outside of my immediate group. I felt embarrassed. I simply could not accept that my husband would deceive me so profoundly. I was obsessed with thoughts about how my life would proceed without him. I didn't let myself think about his angry outbursts, his violent attacks, or our dysfunctional intimate life. I didn't want to accept this as reality. I wanted to hold onto my noble, ethical, gallant husband who stood at the altar watching me walk down the aisle with tears on his face.

I was blind, diabetic, with a kidney transplant, living alone in a house with a guide dog and another pet dog. My life had not been set up for me to live alone with my conditions; Tom handled most things requiring sight. We had moved from our little city home to the suburbs on a wooded lot. I had no means of transportation. I couldn't get to work or to a store. I had no idea how to pay the bills. Hell, I didn't know where the bills were. I didn't know how I'd get the snow blown off the driveway or which company serviced our refrigerator when it broke the next week. The person I loved more than anyone in the world had abandoned me.

He left me for a woman he'd known for a handful of months. I didn't know where my anger was, but I was certainly not aware of it. Instead, my thoughts were stuck on my incredulity that my husband was a philanderer, a cheat. I refused to accept the truth. *Things like this don't happen to me; I'm not a quitter, so our marriage shouldn't break down, either.*

Nights ran into days without sleep. I went to work and lay on the floor of my locked office crying. I barely ate. I was despondent. I spent every day alone and isolated in my house. I simply couldn't see a way out of this pain that ripped into my soul, repeatedly tearing me open. I remembered what I once said to a friend of mine as we talked about the challenges life holds for everyone. "Dying is easy for me; staying alive is the hard part."

Sitting frail and ruined, a shadow of the woman I once was, I knew how to stop the pain.

I went to my diabetic supplies. I drew up an entire syringe of insulin, about fifty times more than normal. Holding the syringe, I plunged the needle deeply into the muscle of my shoulder.

Initially I felt the desperation to correct the low blood sugar, but once I put the insulin into my muscle, the insulin acted very fast. I went to the liquor cabinet and gulped down the contents of whatever bottle my hand found. I went to my bed and sobbed. I pounded my fists on the bed and screamed to the heavens, "Please let me die! I can't bear any more heartache, any more loss and pain in my life." I wailed for everything I'd ever lost, for every prayer unanswered, for every dream smashed to pieces. I was inconsolable.

Exhausted, I lay whimpering on the bed, hoping my anguish would soon stop. *Please let me out,* I whispered in defeat.

Then I thought of my family, my friends, and of Scott, my only brother, who sacrificed his kidney so I could live. I thought about how devastated my mother would be to have to live without me in her life. I pictured her finding my thirty-three year-old dead body on the bed and the unrelenting grief that would entrap her heart forever.

Seeing this image of my grief-stricken mother, my sadness turned to anger. It filled me with a rage so fiery my body stiffened. "You bastard! You rotten, fucking asshole. You are not going to take my life." I screamed at the top of my lungs, "I hate you! You're a pig, a louse. You deserve whatever hell comes your way!" The anger emerged and I did not hold back, pounding my fists on the bed like a mad woman.

My rage saved me. I drank a bottle of soda and called my mother, telling her to take me to the emergency room. I told her I couldn't get my sugar up. It would be many months before I confessed that I attempted suicide that day. I didn't want anyone to know I was such a weak, miserable failure, believing myself to be a helpless victim who couldn't find the courage to face the truth.

As time went on, I discovered his duplicity, his multiple lies and secrets. The mistress is a woman Tom works with. One of my closest family friends knew about his affair but intentionally hid it from me while completing business deals with Tom and his mistress and also hearing of my devastation. I also learned that a friend of mine had secretly been having phone sex with him for years. Not only had my husband been a liar and a cheat, but my close friends colluded with him. The onslaught of lies and betrayals were so crushing it felt as though the crust of the earth had split open and I had been smashed in the crevasse.

I had managed to survive what felt like a death march in Texas. My brother had sacrificed his kidney so I could live. I had to find *my* warrior again, the one who had the strength to face evil as it walked up my stairs. I had to resurrect the part of me that was still breathing beneath the part of me that had been trampled, crumpled up into what felt like unwanted garbage and left behind.

I found hatred. I found a killer rage in me I didn't know existed. I imagined schemes and plots to physically hurt Tom and his bitch mistress. I couldn't stop brooding. I wanted both of them to hurt as much as they hurt me. No form of torture I contrived felt adequate. I wanted revenge.

One month after I found out about Tom's secrets and about the others in my life who'd betrayed me, I had an affair with a married man. The affair stopped my constant grief, temporarily. I knew it was wrong and in that moment I didn't give a damn. If others could be immoral and reckless, why not me? I wanted the whole world to know that nothing mattered more than my suffering. I also didn't want to feel the pain. It was much easier to live in a fantasy life through the affair than to feel the knife in my back.

Eventually my moral compass returned and through a series of consequences, the affair ended. Once the distraction was gone, I had to return to the truth and the pain I had denied.

It took me two solid years to grieve Tom and the destruction of the dreams I held about him and our marriage. At times I thought I would not survive the grief. I blamed myself over and over, hearing Tom's verbal accusation that "I had ruined his life." I anguished over all the things I thought I should have done that I didn't do, and loathed myself for doing things I did do. Paradoxically, I should have been more independent and less assertive. I should have been willing to engage in his pornographic sexual fantasies. I ought to have needed him less even though at times I was sick and afraid. On the other hand, I should have been strong enough to realize the truth of what I knew was happening, but I lacked the faith and courage to admit that the husband I wanted was not the person he was.

Once the self-blame ran its course, I was filled with a mourning and grief that penetrated into every cell. I lost my first love. He left me with no more regard than what he would have given to a stray cat. I could not fathom his insensitivity for my welfare, all for a mistress at work.

My friends' betrayal was as painful to me as Tom's secrets and infidelities. I toiled over the betrayal of the people I most trusted;

some were intentionally silent while others participated in his double-life. The agony of loss and the anger and humiliation of being willfully deceived and intentionally betrayed by these people fueled my need for revenge. I couldn't imagine what I had ever done to them to deserve their disloyalty and their intentional choice to hurt me. If this is how my closest friends treated me, what could I expect from anyone else?

My best revenge, I found, was to rise up from the ashes like a phoenix and come out even better than I was before--which is exactly what I did. My warrior was back! I had to stop the pity party. I had to get over that I was lied to by my once honorable husband and my friends, and realize that although I'd already had my share of rotten experiences, I wasn't immune to more tragedy. I had to start the healing process of this story. I had to take responsibility for once again making my life what I wanted it to be, despite my injury. No one gets a "fair deal" in this life and by now, I certainly knew this was true.

The process of rising from the ashes required first burning down all that was no longer useful. I had to admit to and feel my shame. I had to accept that I had denied the truth of who Tom had become. I had to own my revenge and my rage. And, I had to accept my own shortcomings. I had to recognize and heal the events of my past that prompted me to live defensively rather than proudly. I had to fess up to my own deception and indiscretion of willingly having an affair with a man who was married. The two years I spent healing was my incineration process for the eventual phoenix rising.

It would have been easiest for me to remain justifiably angry. A lot of people colluded with me, making Tom a son-of-a-bitch and me innocent, which was gratifying for a time. It also held me back from starting to heal this shattering experience.

What betrayal or other injustice has you stuck in justified anger? So long as we maintain the belief that we've been wronged and we want someone, anyone, to bear the blame, we remain victims. Victims are powerless to change, and thus there is no healing. Blame and the desire for revenge are normal initial reactions to injustice. But eventually, the blame has to be burned with our other defense strategies that are no longer helpful.

As we sit in the trap of blame and revenge, our desire for joy and peace recedes. The more energy we give to wanting to get even, the less we have available for rebuilding our own lives.

We need to realize that bad things, scandalous things, happen in life and that we are not immune. We aren't special. We don't get a free pass on tragedy. We have no say in some of the things that happen to us. In my case, I thought I ought to be immune from my husband's infidelity because so many bad things had already happened to me. I was outraged that I had to deal with his intentional actions that hurt me when I was already coping with horrible events that were not controllable.

Before we develop a wiser consciousness, we believe we can demand that people meet our expectations for who they ought to be. While we learn to accept the imperfections and idiosyncrasies of others, we also need to honestly see their intolerable truths and move on.

Are you frantically trying to control the universe and the people around you so that you get the life you dream of and ultimately demand? Do you need to let go of the illusion that if you do all the right things, that your hopes and aspirations will be fulfilled? Who or what do you blame for your sadness, your emptiness, or your unfulfilled life? Do you need to stop trying to mold someone into a perfect character so you can be happy? Is it time to give up the brand of a victim and realize the only way your life is going to change is if you begin to heal your real disappointments by coming to terms with the fact that life is not, never has been, and never will be fair? Accepting this truth is difficult because we have been conditioned to believe otherwise.

Fairness is a kindergarten concept that is re-enforced multiple times during our childhood and adolescence. Then, we become adults and we are expected to shift our expectations of life. We're adults, but our child-conditioning is still alive. This portion of our psyche is called, "child-ego" or "child-consciousness."

We all have child-ego within us. It is the instinct in us that is demanding and irrational; the portion of us that says, "I want what I want and I want it now!" When we heal, we are gradually able to recognize when our child-consciousness is directing our thoughts and beliefs. This portion of our personality isn't bad or wrong, but we need to own it for what it is; an un-healed portion of our mental and emotional being. As we mature and heal this portion of our psyche we develop appropriate emotional responses and beliefs fitting for adults. We understand that healthy people do not hold out demands that life (and people) behave the way we insist.

Whether our wounds are self-inflicted or caused by others, they are all potential opportunities to reunite with grace. I had to repair my self-inflicted wound of actively participating in infidelity. Part of my healing was to write to the wife of the man with whom I had the affair. I apologized for my poor choices and for the grievous emotions I caused her and her family. I owned that my actions were reckless and wrong. It was a hard letter to write. I had met her and her children on occasions. Because I knew them, and they me, I felt an even greater need to own my actions and be accountable to those I had wronged. It was an essential healing step I needed in order to return to my grace.

Do you need to make amends for mistakes you've made? Our admissions are a necessary but forgotten ritual. I'm not referring necessarily to religious confession, but rather openly declaring your mistake directly to the person who you've wronged. This is an especially healing action because it serves both the one who has erred as well as the one who has been offended. When we are able to own our mistakes and authentically apologize, we know that our healthy, adult ego is leading rather than our small, child-self who is afraid and unable to tolerate mistakes—both in the self and others. Healing has happened.

THE HEALING

I believed I would never love again. I believed that loving someone only meant my heart would be susceptible to being crushed again, and what's more, I would not have the ability to tolerate the injury. But it was through my experience of betrayal and injustice that I was able to heal enough to develop an abiding strength in my heart and an ability to forgive unconditionally.

In order for me to live and love fully and freely, I had to forgive Tom, his mistress, and my friends. I had to heal the part that wanted to get even and make all of them suffer as much as I had. My ability to reach this authentic forgiveness lay in my ability to admit the truth.

To rise above the abuse and infidelity, I had to look at myself, my marriage, and Tom with spotless honesty. I had to own my behaviors that eroded the relationship instead of nurtured it. I had to admit that Tom the man was not the charming sixteen-year-old boy I met and fell blissfully in love with. No matter how much I wanted to make him into that earlier version, the truth still remained. He was a man with demons he could not overcome. In time, I realized that his weaknesses didn't make him a monster, but rather, a human being. Instead of hating Tom, I began to have compassion for the components of his character that I know haunted him as well. I'm not justifying or excusing his physical abuse or infidelity. I'm looking at the factors that drove him to such destructive, immoral behaviors that were out of alignment with his true nature.

People aren't born liars and cheats. People who are in their right minds don't wake up in the morning and devise ways of wrecking peoples' lives. Once I understood that Tom didn't do what he did "to me," but rather, fell to his own internal fiend, it was easier to forgive him.

Through my reflective healing process, I came to understand that we all have a devil and an angel inside. In other words, we have an internal saboteur who can jeopardize our good and loving nature. I had fallen to my own fiendish nature by having an affair with someone who was not available. What I learned from having had that experience is that I could either continue to ostracize myself for acting outside my value system when I was weak, or admit my indiscretion, forgive my error, and learn from the experience. I realized that I didn't like who I was when I let my dark side overtake my light side. So, I purposefully became cognizant of the various ways my internal devil wanted to sneak out and as best I could, kept that part of me restrained while I made choices that were in alignment with my values. Are you aware of your internal villain and angel? Are you able to admit to the part of you that is capable of destructive thoughts and behaviors? You might not have it in you to physically abuse someone or to have an illicit affair, but maybe your saboteur is alcohol, jealousy, criticizing people who have different values than yours, or other destructive thoughts and behaviors. Maybe you've held a long-standing grievance that overshadows your angelic side.

The choice I made to forgive Tom was ultimately for me. In my healing process, I came to realize that it's impossible to close my heart to one person while keeping it open for others. I don't have to love everyone, but I *choose* love and forgiveness. When I do, my heart opens and I experience more love coming to me and through me. I also knew that whether I chose to hate Tom or to forgive him would influence how I told my story forever.

When I looked honestly at our marriage, Tom did me a big favor. He released me from a caustic and dysfunctional relationship. The grief I experienced from being betrayed by those whom I trusted the most taught me that my heart can get hurt and I can still recover.

I'm not immune from future betrayals or injuries to my heart. If I'm willing to open my heart to love, I must also be willing to open myself to the possibility of future disappointments. People are imperfect; love is always a risk. Yet I choose love instead of a lonely life with a closed heart, detached from self and others, stewing in cynicism. My future heartbreak becomes a rock on which I can stand, because once a heart is broken, it becomes a stronger heart.

I realized that if I were to wait for people to think and behave perfectly before I would consider them as friends, I'd be waiting a long time. My forgiveness of my friends, and even Tom, was born of my own need to be forgiven. I've done things and thought things in the past that I'm not proud of. I hope that I don't have to pay for those decisions for the rest of my life. The forgiveness I extend to others is a bridge that always leads me to self-forgiveness. I can forgive others and adjust my relationship with them based on the level of safety and trust I feel. I learned this was an important step in forgiveness. Some people I may never talk with again. That's not meant as a righteous act or punishment. It's a decision I make so that I have healthy, appropriate relationships. Whether I forgive and continue the same degree of companionship or bless the other and travel on, the essential element for me is that I release them from my vengeful thoughts. I know I've forgiven someone when I have given up the need to get even and when the urge to speak negatively about him or her is gone. So long as I hear myself casting aspersions, I know I'm not healed in this area. Pardoning someone is more powerful than hating them forever.

The degree to which you will be forgiven is the degree to which you forgive others as you heal. You have the strength to own your human imperfection and treat it compassionately. You are capable of realizing the ways in which you neglect instead of nurture others. It is in you to forgive and offer this graciously. Your love is needed and necessary in the world. Your heartaches will heal and your love cannot be destroyed, for you are Love itself.

"When a great injury is done us,
we never recover until we forgive."

Alan Paton

"People are illogical, unreasonable and self-centered.
Love them anyway."

Kent. M. Keith

"The truth is, unless you let go, unless you forgive yourself,
unless you forgive the situation, unless you realize that the
situation is over, you cannot move forward."

Steve Maraboli

"True forgiveness is when you can say,
'Thank you for that experience.'"

Oprah Winfrey

Chapter Six

A GENTLE STRENGTH, AN ENDURING LOVE

I T'S FEBRUARY, 1996. IT'S BEEN EXACTLY TWO YEARS SINCE TOM WALKED out the door and never looked back. I'm at work at the hospital. It's a busy day and I don't have any patience for things to take more time than is necessary. This is my first mistake, because everything in a blind world takes more time than is necessary, or, I should say, it takes more time than if I were sighted. I'm struggling to do a simple task: to plug a cord into a port on my computer. I can't get it in. I've spent now over six minutes trying to do a job that would have taken me less than two seconds to do when I was sighted. The inefficiency and fumbling enrages me and I aggressively shove the plug into the computer, which I know will break the whole thing--which it does. Great, now I'm at a total standstill. As I wait for the IT person to come to make the repair, I pass time on the phone telling a friend about a funny moment that happened over the weekend. As I talk, an energy washes over me from behind. It's coming from the hallway. I turn, letting whoever is there know he can approach me, but no one knocks on the open door, so I continue my story. Again the energy moves into my office, traveling down my body like a breeze from my head, coming to rest at the middle of my back. The sensation, while gentle, is overtly obvious. I turn again – nothing. I finally say, "Is there someone here who needs me?"

Brent steps onto the threshold. "Yes, I'm from IT. I'm here to repair your computer." Hanging up the phone, I swivel in my chair to face him.

My heart expands and a warm flush fills my chest as we face one another. *Something is going on here,* I think. Smiling at him, I say, "You could have knocked or said something. You didn't need to wait around for me to chat on the phone."

Brent replies in an even-tempo, "You were having a good time. I didn't want to interrupt that. Besides, the story you were telling was funny. I'm pretty patient."

The connection between us is instantaneous. He spends less than thirty minutes fixing my computer. I'm observing everything I can about him. I'm curious about him and the cool, calm way he goes about his work. I have to know if he is married. Since I can't see whether or not he is wearing a ring, I have to devise some other way to get my information without being blatantly obvious. It's close to Valentine's Day. I casually ask, "Did you get your sweetie a Valentine?"

"Yes, I'm giving her a mink teddy bear."

Too bad he's taken, I muse, *A mink Teddy bear is a pretty romantic gift.* The mink bears are what actually brought us together. After Brent finished his work in my office that day, our paths didn't cross again for several weeks.

If I couldn't have him, I decided I could have a mink teddy bear. I contacted Brent's mother, the bear creator, and began selling mink bears to the nurses at work. In mid-May, Brent knocked on my office door to drop off some teddy bears his mom had asked him to bring to me. "Remember me?" he asks, and we began a conversation. Since our initial meeting, Brent had discovered his wife was having an affair. When he realized it, he immediately moved out of his home and ended the relationship. Brent cannot abide infidelity.

I'm a volunteer peer counselor working with people about relationships and divorce. I share this with Brent and he comes to see me. I counsel him about repairing his marriage. Despite my efforts to encourage him toward reconciliation, he's already made up his mind. Ethically he cannot return to someone who has betrayed him. I understand and can relate all too well. After some time, our peer talks move to friend talks. It's obvious we are attracted to one another. I'm scared. I'm not about to date a man who's just getting out of a marriage. No way. He seems genuine, but how genuine can a guy be who just found out his wife has been sleeping with another man? I have no interest in being the rebound girl.

We get along great and date for a few months, all the while I'm telling him how this relationship won't work and he's refusing to hear my arguments. I realize we are falling in love. Now I'm really worried. On my suggestion, we decide to see a therapist. I'm sure she'll tell him to pull his head out of his ass and for me to run from him as if he were on fire! But the therapist says, "Some people heal from these things more quickly, Shelli."

Okay, fine, but I'm no small task. I'm blind. I have serious diabetes and a transplanted kidney that is starting to show signs of failure. I have multiple special needs that he hasn't encountered before. In addition to all of this is that I'm an intense person; I laugh hard and cry hard, love fiercely and people know when I'm upset. Loving me is easy; living with me can be hard.

As we negotiate our relationship, I make it a requirement that he live with me for at least nine months so he can know what he is getting into.

I love him so much I want to be sure that he isn't making a commitment that turns out to be more than he bargained for. Besides, I don't want anyone telling me I have "ruined his life" again.

I'm also concerned how he will respond to my blindness. My experience with others is that they don't feel comfortable around blind people and err on the side of being overly helpful which makes me feel diminished, or they don't respond in a way that is helpful for me, which leaves me feeling irritated. For example, when I walk into the break room and say, "Where can I sit?" Someone needs to say, "The second chair from the end is open and the spot by the telephone." Instead, people say, "Anywhere you want." Then I try to explain I don't know which chairs are open and someone will tell another person in the room, as if I'm not there, "How about you put her over there?" Then my blindness ignites my pain that I am different and not an equal part of the group.

Interacting with me as a person who is blind seemed second nature to Brent. From the first moment Brent put his hand in mine, our movements were smooth and synchronized. We were like partners who had danced together for years. Maneuvers others found challenging, like assisting me through a doorway into a store, Brent did effortlessly. His calm, gliding way of moving coupled with my confidence in my body came together in a way that put me immediately at ease. I was relieved and surprised by how naturally we moved together, and how easy he made it be. It was a relief to be with Brent's peaceful flow and confidence after the uncertainty and unpredictability of my first marriage.

Generally people get anxiously excited as they watch me doing something: shrieking out, warning me, jumping into my task, infantilizing me. Brent never fell into this habit that I found annoying in others.

I'm scooping ice cream one night on the screen porch. I have two bowls. I've set a napkin on the table on which to lay the scoop when I'm done. Brent calmly allows me to be an adult, serving the ice cream without advice, or shouts of, "You don't have a full scoop." No stress, no tension, and I feel fabulous that he is able to tolerate watching me without needing to intervene. As I finish, I move my hand toward the napkin to set down the scoop. At the precise right time, Brent glides three fingers onto my hand and with the gentleness of a spring rain, eases the scoop over an inch to rest on the napkin. I look up at him delightfully surprised. "How did you know to do it that way?" I ask.

In his mellow manner he says, "You were doing fine. I was just watching. When I noticed it wasn't going to turn out the way you wanted, I decided to step in. You have to let people move in their own way."

My heart sings with pleasure in his confidence and wisdom. I feel thrilled that the fundamental task of interacting with me isn't going to be a deal–breaker.

The year we date is more a test for me than for Brent. I'm the one with reservations, big ones. I'm still recovering from my betrayal. I'm still healing the wounds I have about trust. I can't believe someone would actually choose me to fall in love with from a field of available women. I have serious medical issues that are only bound to become more involved. Although I'm fairly independent related to blindness, living with a person who is blind can be taxing and I know it. If I can't find something in the house, Brent will have to find it for me. He will have to handle all the mail. There are many times in a day when I need to have something read to me: a bottle, a package, washing instructions on a clothing tag. There is no public transportation where we live, so Brent will have to take me most places. I have a system set up so that no one person needs to do everything I can't do, but there is still a lot Brent will need to do, things most thirty-three-year-old men don't do, like tell me if there's a stain in my panties. I lived alone for two years after my separation and divorce, so it's not that I'm totally dependent. Many blind people live alone and function completely independently. And yet there will be things I know he'll need to do for me that require vision. Needing to rely on another person for these very private tasks can be embarrassing and terribly invasive. It leaves me feeling vulnerable in an extreme way that most adults don't experience. When I feel I can trust that the person helping me is genuine, the insult to my autonomy is decreased. I'm feeling as though I can trust Brent in this regard, but I'm not sure how he will feel after doing these routine tasks day after day, year after year.

My biggest fear is that the diabetes will severely limit not only our lives, but my longevity.

Brent's acceptance made it easier for me to relax my defenses about being loved. In the beginning, I wrongly judged his accepting nature as weakness, never having had the experience of a gentle man. I came to learn that his kindness is his strength.

Before we were married, I asked him why he didn't jump ship and run. "Can't you see that I am a house made of sticks in the path of a cyclone?" I asked him. I love him intensely, but I can't figure out why he loves me, a woman who's defective and damaged, at least in my mind.

He responded honestly, "Loving you is a bigger responsibility than loving someone else, Shell. I know that. Am I afraid sometimes? Sure. But I don't want my fear to be bigger than my love." We were sitting on the front steps, his voice soft, his hands gently holding mine. "There's a lot to love about you. I think I'm lucky. You're smart and funny and beautiful. You're exciting and you make me laugh, and bring a lot of goodness to my life." Brent asked his brother his thoughts about marrying me.

Brian replied, "Well, it will be something new every day." And it is!

As I continue to consider the wisdom of starting this relationship, my medical conditions are predominant in my mind. I have serious issues that, although not all-encompassing every day, could suddenly throw our life off track. I question if it's even fair for me to bring Brent into what will surely be a life of difficulties and perils that are uncommon. I know I'm strong enough to handle the events in my life, but I wonder if he is, or if he even wants to. We get the chance to test his strength within a few months.

Brent and I are visiting Scott and his wife, Nancy, in Chicago. We stroll along the Navy Pier and browse the downtown shops. The activity isn't strenuous, but I seem to tire easily. I check my blood sugar to see if that's a possible culprit, nothing out of the ordinary. On one of the days we drive to Indiana to visit the sand dunes of Lake Michigan. Brent and I are running hand-in-hand through the sand, laughing. Suddenly, I get a dull pain in my chest. I sit down in the sand and it quickly goes away. Brent decides we need to get out of the sand where walking is more strenuous, and spend the remaining part of the afternoon resting. When we get back to Minnesota, I visit one of the cardiologists I work with at the hospital.

I undergo a coronary angiogram. The test shows that diabetes has damaged the arteries of my heart. I'm thirty-four years old. I'm pissed off, sad, scared that the disease I so loathe has further destroyed my body. This new complication caused by diabetes is serious. Heart disease is permanent and progressive. Because the arteries of my heart are damaged, there's a good chance that the arteries of my brain, neck, and legs could also be affected. I am way too young to be thinking about amputations or strokes or death because I now have vascular disease, but that's the reality. I hate diabetes! I want to blow it up, set it on fire and bury it under a million tons of stone. I deserve more than this. Brent deserves more than this.

I have three major blockages in one of my arteries. The doctor is able to open the blockages with angioplasty and stents that will hold the artery open. After the procedure, I lay crying in my hospital bed in the coronary intensive care unit. My nurse is my friend. She silently goes about her business seeing that I am stable. Before she departs, she gives my foot a reassuring squeeze. I lay with my thoughts tangled in my mind. I'm afraid for my health and how this new diagnosis will change how I live. I'm worried about how Brent will handle this news. We've dated for just four months. In that time he's had to intervene to save me from low blood sugars, given me IV insulin, endured my emotional changes caused by fluctuating blood sugars and dealt with countless other idiosyncrasies unique to my special needs, not to mention having to work with personality quirks we all have. I'm afraid this major health change will prove that I truly am too much trouble and not worth the risk.

Brent arrives later in the day. He takes my hand and I manage a weak smile. I'm sure he's going to tell me he's sorry, but this is way too much for a man in his early thirties to deal with. I wish I could run away. He's quiet, standing beside the hospital bed. "How are you?" he asks.

"I'm okay," I lie. With trepidation, I ask him if he's afraid.

"Not afraid, only sad this happened to you," he says and leans down to hug me. "You're strong, baby. I love you." I smile deep inside. I love him, too.

Even though he has given me no cause, I'm afraid to let Brent see what I believe are shortcomings and frailties. Tom had convinced me that "I ruined his life." I fear Brent will judge me. I worry that he'll see my limitations as flaws, my special needs as burdens. I'm worried that the constant battle with diabetes will overwhelm him. I'm terrified that he will grow resentful over time about all the things I can't do as a person who is blind and the limitations it will also put on his life. I'm anxious about wearing my insulin pump to bed, and that he'll view me as unattractive or gross. I fear he will see me walking with my guide dog, or with the white cane in the hospital where we both work and he'll feel less a person for choosing me, like he is getting the booby prize. I feel of less value because I can't go to the store and pick out an outfit for him. I can't help him paint a room or take his six-year-old daughter shopping for dresses and headbands. All this and not to mention I'm not a perfect human being. I'm intense and push myself hard. Anyone with me will have to keep up or I'll bowl them over with my gusto! I focus on all the things I hate in my life and believe he would hate them just as much.

On our very first date I had an incident of drastic low blood sugar; sweat streamed down my face and ran off the tip of my nose. I simultaneously mopped my face with napkins as I poured packets of sugar down my throat. I was horrified having him see me this way as we sat in the booth at the restaurant. Brent never flinched, only asked what he should do and then did it. I was truly shocked at how calm he was, and still is, about all the things I see as intolerable.

As we date, I can see that my welfare is one of Brent's highest priorities. This is hard for me to understand. Growing up, I felt the needs and the wishes of others often seemed to come before mine. I had to learn what it was like to be prioritized in a relationship and how to accept that there wasn't an ulterior motive. Brent considers how his decisions will affect me, but he isn't a martyr.

My friend Theresa, Brent, and I are driving down a city parkway one beautiful summer evening. Brent and I have been dating a little over a month. Theresa is in the back seat. I'm feeling insecure and speak haughtily. I want Brent to know that I've dated other men and they were screw-ups. I have more self-respect than to allow myself to be mistreated again. I look at Brent and with an air of righteousness say, "So, you better just toe the line."

Very deliberately, Brent pulls the car to the side of the road and slowly eases it to a stop. He leisurely turns to look at me, his energy even and calm. In a quiet, controlled voice he says to me, "Wait a minute, here. I'd better toe the line? So far as I can tell, these other guys are the issue, not me. I think you'd better be sure who you're talking to."

I'm beginning to realize Brent is a man who has a lot of power, but doesn't use force to show it. What a difference from Tom's screaming and pushing. I turn in my seat to grin at Theresa, who gives me a high-five. We both know he just sealed the deal! I love this guy more every day!

After a year of watching for signs of his failure and wrestling with my own insecurities, I agree to marry him. Although I have no doubt of Brent's redeeming qualities, I hold on to my reservations about how my medical issues could erode those qualities over time. I question how we will navigate not only daily life, but a multitude of potential, long-term, and perhaps permanent, issues. The love we feel for one another is steamy, but I'm experienced enough to know that daily pressures put out the passion of love too often. A part of me feels I've somehow stolen a valuable commodity that ought to be given to someone with less risk than me. There aren't that many quality men. In the quiet times, my doubtful, frightened thoughts subside and I'm able to see my value. I know that I am more than any illness that happens to be present in me.

JUNE 1997

I'm sitting with Brent on the front deck of our home. Our wedding day is less than a month away. I'm constricted with a gripping fear and shameful embarrassment. I've intentionally deceived him, the one person I love with all my heart. He's been compassionate and understanding of all my physical limitations. He's been patient with my insecurities related to trust and commitment, and I've repaid his trust by hiding the truth from him. Salty tears slide down my cheeks and words choke in my narrowed throat. Each time I attempt my confession, I stop, look down, and hold his hands more tightly. I'm certain he will find what I'm about to expose revolting. I wish I could just go on with the pretense I've created, but I have to tell him. We're going to be married and he will have to know the truth sooner or later.

I gather all the courage I have and say, "I have to tell you something. I've lied to you." He reassures me by stroking my hands and running his finger up my cheek, catching my tears. Minutes go by as I hold the deception inside. I'm scared. What will his reaction be when he learns the truth?

"I should have told you sooner, but I was too afraid," I mutter.

Brent says tenderly, "You can tell me anything, baby. I love you."

His words make me cry harder and feel even more ridiculous. He sits patiently in the space of silence that passes as I continue to feel my humiliation and resist exposing the truth about me. I'm a fraud, at least that's what I think of myself. Interrupting the silence, Brent says, "Is it about your eyes?"

My head snaps up, my back stiffens, and my face changes from guilt to surprise. "What? You know!" I say in shock.

He softly grins at me. "I've known since last fall. I saw your eyes on the nightstand."

I'm shocked to think he knew for months and never said anything. "Why didn't you say something?" I ask.

"I didn't think it was worth mentioning. I knew you'd tell me when you felt it was the right time."

My quandary that day was that I hadn't told Brent that I wear bilateral shells over my real eyes. My real eyes are not equally proportioned and the shells are cosmetic. I take them out at night, like contacts, and my native eyes are beneath them. I had been sneaking around for months, only taking the shells out after we were going to sleep. For the months we had dated Brent continuously commented on my beautiful eyes, even looking into them and describing the intricacies of the colors in them that he loved. These moments were so touching and tender, letting us both feel the love we felt for one another. I couldn't bring myself to break the spell by saying, "Thanks. They're fake."

My eyes are a symbol of a lot of pain for me. Before I lost my eyesight, my eyes were the one attribute I felt confident about. I could look into a mirror and gaze at my eyes for long periods of time, luxuriating in the depth I saw in them. Mystics say that the eyes are the doorway to the soul. But not for me; mine are painted plastic material. Making eye contact is one of the most profound emotional experiences people have. We feel most seen through direct eye contact. Since Brent always commented on my eyes, I think that Brent believes he's been seeing my real eyes; that he's been looking into my soul. I'm afraid that Brent has fallen in love with what he believes is me, but the prosthetics are not me. The fact that he's been gazing into replicas and beneath them my own eyes are shrunken, unequal, distorted, and what I believe is ugly and broken is indescribably sad for me. *Why would someone want to sacrifice the most intensely meaningful experience of seeing a person's soul in exchange for looking at inanimate plastic?* I ask myself.

My secret revealed, I hide my face in embarrassment in his chest and weep. He rubs my back slowly. "Don't worry about silly things like that, baby," Brent reassures me.

"Doesn't it bother you?" I ask him.

He responds gently, "Why would something like that bother me? It doesn't define who you are. It's not part of your character, is it? I didn't fall in love with your fake eyes or your blind eyes; I fell in love with you."

I'm humbled and awed. This is why I love him so much; he is wise in an ordinary way. I find this characteristic not only reassuring, but also alluring.

I'm standing in a natural alleyway of lilacs wearing a white lace skirt and top purchased from a street vender in Mexico. I have a ring of fresh flowers in my hair and a bunch in my hand. At the front of the aisle, a wooden flute plays and wedding guests stand in a circle anticipating my arrival on my brother's arm.

I arrive at Brent's side and I feel the brilliant sunshine on my face as I smile at him. He tenderly takes my hand in his and gracefully pulls me to his side. "You are beautiful; especially in this moment," he says. My heart melts and I feel secure as he holds me snugly beside him. I'm thinking, *How did I get this lucky? He could have picked anyone.* I still haven't figured him out, but in this moment, my heart, not my head, is the only thing that matters.

Have the voices in your head convinced you that you are too much trouble, that you somehow don't measure up to the next person? You are likely not blind nor have a medical condition that dictates your life, but we all can feel lacking or defective, the last one chosen, in one way or another. The voices that want to keep us small bellow like a horn in the fog. During the healing process we can ferret out the origin of these recriminating voices. Then we can construct healthier thoughts and opinions about ourselves. Once we do, we can then receive the love and approval of which we are all deserving, regardless of our past errors, annoying habits, and imperfections.

THE HEALING

Brent taught me the healing power of unconditional love and the essential characteristics of authentic strength.

I saw myself as unwanted, broken merchandise. I truly believed I was too great a liability, had too many things wrong with me to be chosen as a partner. I felt like the runt of the litter. I believed I was a basically good person with a fun personality, that I was attractive and had a professional occupation. Yet for most of my life I had an internal voice that taunted me, telling me I was too much trouble, a bother, an inconvenience and therefore, undesirable. After my divorce I dated a man who was also vision impaired. Someone very close to me said, "It's bad enough with you, but hauling two of you around is a real pain." I believed my internal mocking voice even more because a key person in my life had told me that being with me was like hauling around a sack of potatoes. His words made me believe Tom was right, my disability, which is a part of me, had ruined his life. I truly was as worthless as the trash.

Then Brent came into my life and he began teaching me what un-conditional love truly means. He was unbiased and saw me as whole, equal to him. He was able to look beyond the hardships and limitations to what a relationship with me would mean. Brent never saw me as an inconvenience. He didn't feel he was hauling me around. His unconditional love comforted me in my self-doubt. He followed his heart and believed in its unfaltering strength. His acceptance of me in all of my beauty and imperfection taught me self-acceptance.

Brent showed me how to be strong without being demanding or manipulative. Through Brent I learned that I had a distorted belief about men and masculinity. I thought that all men were aggressive, domineering, and had unpredictable emotions. And if his emotions changed, it was because of something I did or didn't do. I had concluded that these were quintessential characteristics that defined masculinity. In Brent I learned an entirely different definition of masculinity and strength. I learned that the most relevant characteristic of strength was respectfulness, that true masculinity includes traits like even-temperedness, patience, and strength born of confidence. As a result, I was able to begin to heal my self-protective, controlling habits in my relationships with men and as time went on, I was able to transfer my newfound softness to my other relationships as well.

Brent proved to me that I'm worthy of being loved. He taught me that a person of good character can value love more than self-absorption. Brent taught me that one of the key qualities to seek out in a relationship is kindness. I hadn't learned this before. I had been focused on fascination, brawn, sex appeal and influence. Kindness is the characteristic, however, that will sustain a relationship when intrigue and vivaciousness expire. I wanted to claim this noble characteristic for myself as well. I watched Brent engage in life with few demands that others be the way he wanted them to be. Brent was kind and accepted me for the person I was. I began to follow his example and became conscious of how often I overtly or covertly demanded others meet my expectations.

I began to realize that my demands were motivated by unmet needs from my childhood. If I demanded that others prioritize my needs above theirs, my real need was that I yearned to have my needs be seen as important when I was young. Or if I demanded that people always do things the way I wanted them done, my real need was that I wanted to have a voice in events that affected me in my earlier life. To heal my sometimes demanding nature, I had to understand that the fuel for my demand had nothing to do with the present moment. I had to find my real unmet needs from earlier in my life and feel the distress from that time so I could release it. When I did, the urge to be demanding today nearly disappeared, and I discovered that those demands had never given me comfort in the first place.

I was able to begin to heal my suspicion of betrayal. I have enduring trust in Brent. His dedication and devotion to me, and the vows of commitment we took have reinforced my faith in the possibility that fidelity is sustainable and that love, when given with unconditional kindness, is the eternal abiding goodness in the world.

We create dreams for our lives and we set our hearts on them. We make plans and feel invincible, trusting that our hopes will bear fruit and life will unfold in a glorious way. If we are blessed, some of these aspirations ripen. Others wither on the vine. What dream of yours crashed against the rocks and now is irretrievable? Have you felt so undermined, so deceived, that you have abandoned the idea of trusting, loving, or ever taking a risk again? As you bear witness to your own life, are you transferring painful messages you heard earlier onto the tongue of another? You may feel that life is only for the lucky, the special people, the gifted, and the beautiful. I spent a long while feeling I had to be perfect in order to be loved. Then I healed enough to believe in myself. I was able to focus on all the exceptional things about me, or the things that simply made me average. Perpetual self-criticism was both unattractive and ultimately drained my energy.

Is your self-worth linked to the typical cultural good/bad, honor/ shame system that has dominated our beliefs for hundreds of years?

That system is called duality, wherein identity is split, and I can only be one and not the other: where I'm either successful and wonderful or I'm a failure and shameful. This system is based on external factors rather than an internal understanding and acceptance of the self as being divinely created.

This dualistic system is primarily based on external comparisons. We see this recorded in the Hebrew bible in the story of Cain and Abel: two brothers' achievements being compared, one favorably and the other unfavorably. Tragically, the external comparison created such anguish and shame that a brother is driven to murder. Whether the story happened just this way or is an allegory, it is illustrative of how external comparisons drive the human ego toward jealousy, envy, separation from others, and the need to somehow pacify our ego's need for validation through achieving more or through revenge.

Today we continue to look outside for validation, and it generally doesn't satisfy our insecurity. We compare our level of education against others, our physical abilities, what we have acquired, everything. You get the picture. Comparison is normal in a world that promotes and encourages external accomplishments as the quintessential indicator of worth. However, these external validators are not enduring; that's why we require them over and over again. Our worthiness comes from our Divinity, not what we've acquired nor accomplished.

Father Richard Rohr writes about healing dualistic thinking and his theories often match my own. Fr. Rohr speaks of the "contemplative mind." I use the term "consciousness." As we heal our dualistic thinking, we are able to move into what Fr. Rohr calls "the contemplative mind." This system could care less what the rest of the world is doing or achieving. It focuses on the individual and is a solitary, internal process. Instead of asking ourselves, *Am I good enough? Am I normal?* the process brings the individual inward and asks questions such as, *What are my values? How am I doing at living those values? What things in my own thinking or in my past experiences ignite my shame? How can I return to inner peace?* Once we begin to seek conscious living through the contemplative mind, we quiet our perpetual need to compete and to compare. Our anxiety decreases and we feel enduring fulfillment. Learning this process is what I call, "Living With Consciousness™," and is a step-by-step process that actually works.

As we heal our stories, we are drawn to internal reflection. The process leaves us with unshakable satisfaction and composure regardless of what current societal norms label as proper achievements. Leaning on our internal identity relieves us of external pressures to achieve more, have more, in order to feel worthy. This is not to say that accomplishment is inherently wrong or bad. Rather it's about the purpose, or intention, of our striving, and only the individual can honestly know what that is.

If others have teased, mocked, or criticized you, you likely have internalized those words and believed them. This is a perfect set up for the comparative and competitive dualistic system in our culture. With time and persistence in the healing process, we begin to see the Self as sacred and worthy of love and respect. Shifting from the external system to an internal process of worthiness gives us the tenaciousness to form new dreams and open our hearts to love.

My first love wasn't the prince I contrived him to be. My fairy tale ended. I could have remained hopelessly lost in the enchanted forest. Had I done so, I would have missed the gift of Brent and all the lessons of sustainable love he taught me.

Dreams sometimes tear apart. Our healing task is to learn from these experiences, learn what to do differently next time, develop resiliency, and dare to conceive new dreams. New dreams aren't second-best. They are the indicators of a fertile and trusting spirit that above all else, believes and hopes eternally. Are you aware of your own resistance to making new dreams because you feel betrayed or disillusioned? Or because you can't fathom that another dream will ever be as good? Is it time for you to rise like the phoenix and start anew?

No dream lasts forever; they all have natural conclusions. When dreams end, we can feel just as lost and hurt as we do when a dream breaks.

Children grow up and move away. Beloved pets die. People we love take their final breaths, leaving us here without them. We age. Our youthful agility recedes and so our brisk morning run becomes a short stroll. The cabin at the lake stands solemnly silent, the playhouse and swing set no longer used. Our sizzling summer parties dwindle, replaced by frosty winters and what was new and intriguing becomes drab. We reminisce about the old days when love and life were young and strong.

We feel the absence of dreams that have peaked and we wonder how to fill the void. These are the normal endings in life we wish we didn't have to accept. They can leave us feeling downhearted, lonely, and even depressed, because when a dream dies so does the era when it was born. We often feel hollow and desolate because we can't go back and live it all over again. Our grief is great at these times because not only is the dream gone, but who we were in that time and with those people in those dreams are also gone. It's essential we honor the emotions we feel at these times rather than waving them away saying, *This is just part of life.* What era of your past and the vibrancy of that period have been lain to rest? What aspects of you have vanished with the passing of a loved one, your vibrant body, or your expired dream? Have you honored your emotions related to these normal losses?

When dreams reach their natural sunset it's just as important to foster new dreams as it is when a dream breaks. We need to embrace and welcome the next era of life and the new opportunities therein. Our goals and ambitions need to continuously evolve as we mature and our lives change. To entrench ourselves in the past is to kill the innate desire of the spirit to create, to expand, and to be engaged with the present. This is how the soul continues to express its longings rather than becoming brittle and withered.

Everyone gets knocked down or falls down. Decide that you're capable of standing up as many times as necessary. New dreams and new loves are within your reach. Appreciate the power spawned of gentleness. Seek the one who is kind. Feel worthy of tenderness, respect, and love that ignite your passion. *Be* the love you wish to receive and welcome it when it arrives.

"Your task is not to seek for love,
but merely to seek and find all the barriers
within yourself that you have built against it."

Rumi

"Love is what heals the personality. There is nothing that cannot be healed by love. There is nothing but love."

Gary Zukav

"The purpose of relationship is not to have another who might complete you, but to have another with whom you might share your completeness."

Neale Donald Walsch

"Sometimes the heart sees what is invisible to the eyes."

Jackson Brown

""You have to keep breaking your heart until it opens."

Rumi

Chapter Seven

THE COMPLICATED HARMONY OF GIVING AND RECEIVING

PART I

IN THE SUMMER OF 2007 MY NEPHROLOGIST ADVISED ME TO MEET with the transplant team at the University of Minnesota to talk about the necessity for another kidney transplant. My kidney from Scott was showing signs of failure. I'd kept it going by having many invasive procedures. I was doing okay at the moment, but the kidney doctor knew that I would soon need another organ to stay alive, or at the very least to avoid dialysis.

Almost a year later I'm asleep in my bed at home. The phone rings, startling me awake. It's a transplant surgeon at the University calling. "We have a possible organ for you." I sit up as I try to get my brain to understand what my ears heard. I hit the button on the audible clock on the night-stand beside my bed. It's 12:15 AM on June 4, 2008—the precise date that my first kidney transplant was scheduled in 1987. "What is it?" I ask the doctor. "It's a kidney–pancreas offer," the doctor says. His English is heavily accented. "A kidney and pancreas?" I ask bewildered. I'm waiting for just a pancreas offer; I already have a living kidney donor who has been waiting for six weeks for a pancreas offer to come through so we can do the double transplant. "The offer is both the kidney and the pancreas. You'd have to take both organs. And, it's a DCD," the heavily accented voice tells me in a rushed manner.

I'm inundated with emotion and confused; my mind is spinning. A surge of adrenaline rushes through my body making my heart race and my muscles stiffen. It's hard for me to take a breath. "Wait, slow down. What's a DCD?" I say with emphasis on "DCD." I've never heard this term before.

The doctor explains that the offer is from a fifteen-year-old girl. My stomach flips and my heart falls to my feet- a child. "DCD means donation after cardiac death." He explains that this means that the girl is still on life support and the medical team is unsure if her heart will stop once she is taken off the machines. I'm listening to a doctor that I don't know explain to me the particulars about a fifteen-year-old girl who is likely going to die and how I could have her organs. I'm not at all prepared for this call.

I've been waiting for a call offering only a pancreas. I feel like I'm going to pass out. The doctor says they will call me in a few more hours when they know more about the donor, but I shouldn't have anything to eat until they call me. He says, "Go back to sleep." The whole phone call takes no more than eight minutes. Setting the phone in the cradle, my thoughts a jumbled mess, I think, *Sure, just go back to sleep.*

I don't go back to sleep. Instead, I wake Brent and explain what just happened. We look at one another, the questions in our minds hanging unspoken between us: Where's my single pancreas offer? What about

Jason who has been waiting to donate his kidney to me? Should I take this offer? How good is the match? And why am I getting an offer for a double organ transplant that will save my life on my forty-sixth birthday, of all days?

THE SUMMER BEFORE.

Brent and I meet with the lead transplant surgeon. He's also one of the pioneers who introduced pancreas transplants. Although I'm meeting the physician to talk about a kidney, the possibility of a pancreas transplant lingers in the far recesses of my mind. A pancreas could mean I wouldn't have diabetes any longer. We are eager for the meeting with him since we know he has decades of experience and hopefully will have good answers to our many questions. The meeting doesn't go as smoothly as we had imagined it would.

He explains to us that I should find a living donor rather than rely on a cadaver kidney. Living kidneys always last longer and have less possibility for issues after transplant than do those that are called "deceased" organs. He suggests offhandedly that I find a living donor, offhandedly like someone might say, "Get a new hard drive for your computer rather than a refurbished one." We go on with the meeting and we learn more about the kidney transplant details. As he sifts through my chart, he hurriedly looks at me and says with fervor, "Your kidney was in 1987. Why haven't you been back for your pancreas transplant since then?" I'm astonished. He's rattling off questions, statistics, and suggestions to me. I'm a seasoned critical care nurse and I can scarcely keep up with him. Besides, who said I was *supposed* to have a pancreas transplant?

"Look, I haven't even given the idea of a pancreas transplant serious consideration. I'm only here to talk about what I need to do to get a kidney," I retort. I'm annoyed with his cavalier attitude. It might be an everyday thing for him, but the thought of getting a pancreas transplant is only a vague concept in my mind. And truth be told, I'm not even sold on the whole idea of undergoing another kidney transplant at this moment of my life.

Brent and I leave the first meeting with the feeling we have just been to a sales pitch for a timeshare in Mexico. The doctor seems nonchalant about an event that for us is monumental. I have grave reservations about the immune suppression medications I would need to take to prevent my body from rejecting the new organs. Since I have a perfect match with Scott's kidney, I have gotten by with very minimal immune suppressing medications. The new medications would be stronger and have the possibility of many more side effects that frighten me and give me great pause: memory loss, skin cancer, lymphoma, and those not so dastardly but just as upsetting effects such as hair loss and lifelong gastrointestinal issues. Organ transplant is not the happy ending to a sad story. While it is true that the organs extend life to someone who would otherwise die, the complications and medication side effects can be harrowing. The organs can reject at any time after transplant. The truth is, the saga is never over for the organ recipient.

After subsequent appointments with the transplant team at the University, we feel more assured. I accept the truth that my kidney is failing and I'll soon need dialysis without a new, healthy kidney. The point remains that a kidney from a living donor is substantially preferred over a cadaver kidney. I am literally tasked to find someone to donate a kidney to me. Mystified, I ponder how I would even ask someone such a question and under what circumstances. I have difficulty asking people for help with reading a package label; how would I ever ask someone for a kidney?

Although a successful pancreas transplant meant I would be free from diabetes, I have significant trepidation. I'd heard terrible stories about the difficulty recovering from such a surgery, even that people die from incisional infection after a pancreas transplant. On the other hand, diabetes is killing me. The perpetual fluctuations of my blood sugars rules our lives. Diabetes has already damaged Scott's kidney as well as my own kidneys. Diabetes cost me my eyesight. It's already created heart and vascular disease in my middle-age body. Before my first kidney transplant, diabetes damaged the nerves of my stomach, giving me a condition called, "gastroparesis." This condition created most of the vomiting before my first transplant. Thankfully, this condition improved after the first transplant. But it can return any time as long as diabetes strafes my body.

Brent has rescued me from death too many times. After getting clarification about the dreadful rumors I have heard, I decided the risk of the pancreas was a better risk than continuing to live with diabetes. The pancreas, however, would need to come from a cadaver. The doctors explain that my best outcome will be to have one surgery: a double organ transplant. This means that my living kidney donor will have to agree to emergency surgery, so the kidney will be available the moment a pancreas offer is made. Although I've already been through one kidney transplant, that was a scheduled operation. I was very ill when I had the first transplant. While I am not currently critically ill, my overall health is worse from the years of additional damage caused by diabetes. I have seven stents in my heart and my blood pressure is high. I have kidney failure and severe diabetes. It's terrifying to think about my surgical risk.

Brent is immediately tested to see if his kidney would match. Two girlfriends also offer to be my donor and are tested. These options don't work out. One day Brent is talking at work with one of his co-workers. He tells her that the surgeon instructed me to find a person to donate on my behalf. From across the room, a third co-worker says, "I'll do that." It was Jason. Brent had recently started working with him and they had quickly become friends. I didn't know him at all. If Jason matches, he has two stipulations: the surgery will have to take place outside of hockey season so he can continue playing as the goalie on his city team. And, since Jason has no family members in Minnesota, his mother needs to be flown here from Pennsylvania to be here for the surgery. Jason is tested and he is a match.

Remarkably, I have found the living donor the surgeon instructed me to find in only a couple of months! Hockey season is just starting. We decide to plan for a surgery in the spring, after the season is over. I am put on a waiting list for a cadaver pancreas, but in what's known as "inactive" status. Accruing time on the list moves me higher up on the list, but if a match comes through, I will not be offered the organ until I move to active status.

Even though I have the living donor for the kidney, I learn that I will be put on three different donation lists to ensure my best outcome. My name is put on the pancreas only, kidney only, and both pancreas and kidney lists. While I understand the concept of putting me on three different lists, I also feel confused. Why is the surgeon so emphatic about finding a living donor if I have been put on lists that will offer me a cadaver kidney? It's explained to me that I can possibly get an offer from someone who is a better match for me than Jason, which decreases the possibility of my body rejecting the organs. The system of organ donation is nationally orchestrated and is extremely complex and highly sophisticated.

As I progress in this journey, I am grateful I am a registered nurse; at least I understand the language and rationale being used. Just the same, I often feel deluged by many variables that seemed to change frequently. Everyone involved is also uniquely affected.

Over the winter and spring, Jason and I get to know one another. We talk about why he would do such a thing – offer his kidney to a stranger. He says he doesn't really know why, but has always known he would be destined to donate, for some inexplicable reason. Jason previously saw a story on the news about a child who needed a kidney. After seeing the story, Jason went to be tested to see if he matched the child, but he didn't. We talk about how his mother and family would get here in time for the emergency surgery. I consult with the team at the University. They tell me that since I have been accruing time for so long, I will be very high on the list. This makes it likely that a pancreas offer will be made quite quickly after we move to active status. I am told that I might expect several offers as I have the most common blood type and I have no antibodies that prevent me from taking any offer. I am also told that when an offer is made, there is generally at least twelve hours and up to twenty-four hours before surgery. Given this information, we decide that we will fly Jason's Mom here once we are on active status and then get the rest of the family here on an emergent basis once we know that surgery is upon us. This plan seems logical and feasible months before surgery, but it doesn't work out to be.

Jason's hockey season is set to end on April 16. We decide to move to active status on that date, which means I can get a call at any hour of any day, starting that very day. As April arrives, we all become more excited and more anxious. I am going to get a life-saving kidney from Jason and a life-changing pancreas from a stranger.

I spend hours trying to fathom what my life will be like free from diabetes. Each time I test my blood sugar or give insulin through my pump, I consider what it will be like to have my body work like everyone else's. Every time I suck down boxes of juice to remedy the confusion and weakness of my low blood sugar, I think about never needing to do this again. I envision what it will be like to be free of the relentless concern that Brent will find me in a semi-conscious state. I'm retaining fluid and my labs are showing that my kidney is struggling more. I'm having an invasive procedure every other month to put a plastic tube in the ureter to keep it open. My body negatively reacts to the necessary material and I develop a systemic candida infection. Yeast is growing in and on my body. I have to take very strong medicine that makes me feel even more sick. I know if I don't get a kidney soon I will need to be on dialysis. Recalling my wretched experience with dialysis so many years ago in Texas, I shudder at the thought of that misery again. I am scared but more than this I'm eagerly anticipating a surgery that I hope will lead to a resurrection of my physical, emotional, and spiritual life.

I believe everything is all set and in order, but just two weeks before our active date, the tides suddenly turn. I wonder if I will have a nervous breakdown.

I don't know how or when Jason told his family about his decision to donate a kidney. After being on the waiting list for over eight months, two weeks before I am about to move to active status, I receive a late night e-mail from his father, whom I had never before spoken with. The note is blunt; his questions and narrative are totally unanticipated. I am stunned. As I take in all he has written, I feel as though I have done something wrong and have to defend the fact that I am sick and will die without a kidney. Although his note doesn't say it outright, I know he is scared for his son and has legitimate concerns. However, I am not the person to be asking these questions of. I am the sick one. I didn't ask Jason for his kidney; he offered it.

My mind spins with fear, *Why didn't Jason's dad ask these questions months ago?* The donor program has nurses and social workers and doctors who handle all of the questions of the donors and families. I put my face in my hands and bawl. Shaking, I rush to Brent's side. Brent reassures me that Jason will handle his family.

I go to bed that night filled with anguish, worry, and uncertainty. I feel the terrible truth that I am at the mercy of Jason and the strength of his conviction in his decision. The truth makes me feel helpless and dependent and vulnerable in a way I haven't felt before. I hate knowing that I am powerless to do anything. Equally, I hate the feeling that I am the cause of any strife in Jason's family. I personalize the entire matter.

Brent is right; Jason does handle his family's concerns.

On April 16, 2008, I am moved to active status. All of us: me, Brent, Jason, my parents, Jason's parents are instantly filled with excitement laced with anxiety. Since I am high on the list, the call can come any time. It is impossible not to dwell on when it will happen.

We get together with Jason and his mom often, offering our support to both of them and huddling together in our effort to change my life. We feel like a cohesive team pushing toward a goal. I check in with Jason frequently, making sure he is still onboard. He remains steadfast.

We wait. And wait. And wait. I carry my cell phone day and night. The waiting is excruciating. I feel like I'm holding my breath all day, every day. I'm filled with the urge to rush repeatedly to check my position on the list, which is an arbitrary position. I want something to relax my constantly tense nerves. But all I can do is wait for the phone to ring. I have no control over what offers will be made or when. I feel powerless, and I am. Everyone's life is literally on hold as the hours tick off and the days go by. It's agonizing. And there's not one damn thing I can do about it.

The phone rings in my **office**. It's April 22nd. I listen to my nurse coordinator give me the details of my first offer. It is for both a kidney and pancreas. What? I'm expecting a pancreas-only offer. I'm totally caught off-guard. My coordinator reminds me that my name is on three different donation lists. My mind is bombarded. I can ask a few questions about the donor, but at this moment, sitting at work thinking I'm going to have an ordinary day, any sensible question eludes me. My brain finally engages and I'm able to ask a couple key questions.

Trembling with anxiety, I tell the coordinator I'll call her back. I'm too nervous; my mind can't process. I page my best friend at work, Amy, another nurse at the hospital, and get her to come to my office immediately to help me sort all this out. This is the most stressful, pressure-filled situation I've ever been in. In less than five minutes an offer is made and I'm expected to instantaneously make a decision. In that time I'm supposed to say yes or no to an organ that is going to be part of my body forever. Most people take weeks or months to decide about a car they'll drive for a few years and here I am making decisions about permanent body parts over the phone in a matter of minutes. It seems hideously insane to me. My heart is racing as I consider this offer. With Amy's help, I decide to turn down the offer based on the donor's medical history. I call the coordinator back and decline. Then I go to the bathroom and throw up.

One week later I have another offer for a pancreas only. It is from a man with a long history of daily alcohol use. Although I know Jason is waiting with his mother here, displaced from her home and husband, I have to decline. I feel sick to my stomach again. I call Jason and tell him about the offer and my decline. He assures me he and his mother are fine. He says I have to think about what is best for me.

Thinking about only me is impossible. I have Jason and his whole family on hold. My family is tense. Brent is filled with apprehension that I'll make a decision that is best for Jason and not me. I've never felt so much pressure and fear that I'll make the wrong decision. I can't sleep or eat. I can't talk about it, and I can't not talk about it. I find myself once again facing the truth that I am mostly a passive player in determining my fate. I am incapable of making pancreas offers materialize, and I can only receive a pancreas if I have the extraordinarily gracious gift of Jason's kidney.

The whole month of May passes without the phone ringing. *Where is my offer they said would come quickly? Have I sabotaged myself by passing up two offers that didn't seem right for me?* At times I want to start walking and simply disappear, leaving behind this chaotic circus that is my life.

I pray ceaselessly. The more the time passes, the more reservations I develop over the pancreas. I have a very difficult time coming to terms with the fact that I am praying for an organ offer, which means I am hoping that a viable person will die. The notion goes against every bit of my values and my heart. I write in my Caring Bridge journal one day, "... In all of this prayer and anxiety, urging the call to come, I'm nagged by the idea that in order for me to get what I need, someone else has to get what they don't want. As my own mother prays at her bedside for my salvation to arrive, another mother also prays for her child's salvation. So, then, what becomes the answer to prayers? Whose prayer will be heard? And whose will be, seemingly, passed over?"

The waiting consumes us. Every time Brent and I hear emergency sirens on the road we wonder, *Will this be my organ offer?* We think thoughts we never considered part of our disposition. We go through the motions of daily living, but an endless anxiety colors everything. My mind returns to the late night e-mail and the idea that Jason's family initially had reservations about all of this. Now the wait is more than I was told. *These people are going to hate me,* I think. I'm tormented from every angle. Life is suspended.

On my birthday, the call comes in the middle of the night for the pancreas–kidney offer from the fifteen-year-old girl. It is very upsetting. Although I'm getting an offer, it's not the pancreas-only offer I've planned for. I'm sickened. Taking this offer means I'll have to call Jason and say, *Never mind! You and your family have been waiting for six weeks but I've decided to take a different offer.* How can I be so selfish and manipulative of others' lives? My mind races. What about the surgeon's advice to find a living kidney donor? How can I know what the right decision is? It seems every answer only leads me into more questions. I go to work. I talk with Brent, Mom, and my critical care nurse friends. Of course, no one has any more wisdom than do I. After hours of distraught deliberation, two transplant surgeons call me from the University. In general, it is against policy to advise a recipient whether to take an offer or not. But they bend the rules. They tell me, "You'd be a fool not to take this offer."

With a heavy sigh, I sit down in the chair in my office. I have to trust that if Jason is the kind of man who would offer to donate his kidney so I could live, he will be able to accept that this offer appears to be my best chance. I take the offer. Then I make the hardest call I hope I ever have to make and tell Jason my decision. Hearing his disappointment makes me feel like a traitor. I sit weeping behind the closed door of my office. My friend Cindy comes to see me. She says, "You need to focus on the fact that you are the sick one here, Shelli. You have to trust that Jason can take care of himself. You need to get yourself ready to have a double organ transplant in a matter of hours." I know she's right. I'm besieged by my emotions. There's so much to think about and respond to. My hands run nervously through my hair. I take a deep breath and refocus. Brent comes to my office, takes my hand in his and we leave.

I pack a suitcase for my anticipated two-to-three week stay at the hospital. Brent and I pick up Mom and Brent's sister joins us. We meet with the transplant surgeon at the University. He says that the family of the donor will take her off life support late in the afternoon when all of her family can be there. The surgeon explains that if the girl's heart doesn't stop beating within forty-five minutes after she's removed from life support, I won't get the organs. We learn that the girl is right here in Minneapolis, which makes her organs as close to 'living' as is possible from a cadaver.

I'm waiting, knowing that a fifteen–year–old child's family is gathering to say their final good-byes. I'm sitting with my own family on the patio of a restaurant on the university campus. People are walking their dogs; skateboarders are whizzing by. It's my forty-sixth birthday and I'm waiting for a child to take her final breath so I can hope to start a new life of my own. My mind reels. I'm torn between my own life and this young girl's. Then my thoughts turn to Jason sitting in his apartment with his mother and not with us as we've planned for months. A deluge of emotions falls unorganized through me. The story I'm living is getting more insane. I no longer know what to feel or what to pray for, so I choose to pray for peace, which comes, but only for a moment.

Sitting on the patio of the restaurant, my cell phone rings. The rest of my family is eating. I've been instructed not to eat or drink anything in anticipation of the surgery. I answer the phone on the first ring. My family looks at me in silent expectation. "It's a no-go," the doctor on the phone says. "We will try again another time." I say, "I understand." He hangs up and I'm left holding my phone. The call takes no more than twenty seconds. I look at my family and say, "She didn't die in time. Game over. Let's go home." I stand up, pushing my patio chair away and reach for Brent's hand to guide me down the street. My mother is aghast. In shocked silence we walk to our cars. I go home and sit numbly at my computer. I have to update my Caring Bridge journal that told hundreds of people I was going to the hospital. After months of preparation, I'm dismissed in a nanosecond. I'm emotionally bankrupt. I don't think human beings are designed to cope with this kind of upheaval; I'm certainly not. Sitting at my desk, the evening turns to night and I haven't written a word. I'm utterly hollow.

Jason is now back on-deck to be the donor. It feels inhumane. The entire ordeal is wearing on Jason and his mother, who has left her husband in Pennsylvania to live with Jason for almost eight weeks. I understand their frustration. Jason tells me we have to put an end-date to the wait. I agree and completely understand. Jason says he can't be available after June 30th. I feel shameful as if I had anything to do with the lack of pancreas offers.

Over Memorial weekend we have an honest talk. Jason asks me what I want to do: have a single surgery that gives me his kidney and wait for a pancreas to come later, or stick with our original plan. I hesitate.

Should I lie? Or should I answer him honestly like he asked me to do? I say I'd rather wait because the doctors say one surgery decreases my chances of getting lymphoma from having to take the intense immune suppressants twice. Jason says, "I'm glad you said that, because if you hadn't, I would have said you were lying."

I wish I could rewind the whole year and do it over. Nothing is working out the way it was explained or the way we planned. I'm beginning to let in my old beliefs that a malevolent, heartless God is trying to break me. I'm a healer who talks about faith and surrender and trusting in the universe, but at this moment it is difficult to find a dram of confidence: not in God, medicine, or myself.

Four days later I get a call. It's for a pancreas only. I listen to the details of the offer. Then the doctor says, "You're second in line." What the hell! I've never heard of being first or second in line for an offer. I'm stupefied. *There is a person who's first in line? What sort of game is being played here?* I think. Another man is first in line. He's going to the hospital to have blood drawn right now. If his antibodies match the organ, he gets it. The doctor says he'll call back in a few hours to let me know if I've moved up and should come to the hospital. The hours pass as if an eternity; finally the phone rings. The first person is a match. Now I'm positive I'm being tortured.

The day after the offer I call the surgeon. I feel rocked off my center with the idea that an offer might land me in second place. During the conversation I learn things I've never been told. The doctor says that just because an offer is made, it doesn't mean the organ will be transplanted. Although an organ can be in perfect condition at the time of procurement, because of lack of blood, it can become damaged to the point where it is unusable once it reaches the University. I won't know if the organ will be actually transplanted until I'm at the hospital, prepped and ready for the operating room. I call a friend and say, "I want ten shots of tequila."

On June 20th I'm sitting in our living room waiting to leave for dinner at the home of some friends. I'm not feeling exceptionally well. The kidney failure is causing me to retain a good deal of fluid. I've gained almost twenty-five pounds over the last year. My hands, face and legs are swollen. I'm listening to the beautiful sounds of singing birds through the open windows when the phone rings. I recognize the phone number. Flooded with apprehension, I answer it. "This is transplant at the university. We have a pancreas offer for you." "Am I first? I mean, is it mine?" I ask. "Yes," comes the reply. Now the real journey begins.

The pancreas offer is from a seventeen-year-old girl who had a blood clotting disorder. She suffered a stroke after stopping her blood thinners in preparation for oral surgery. My heart is ripped. Her family's greatest tragedy is my family's greatest miracle. The pancreas offer is spectacular; a high antigen match, young and viable, no significant health history. I can once again feel the Divine plan at work. From a place deep within my soul I know all of the agonizing days behind me have been purposed to bring me to this precise Divine moment.

All of us are told to come to the hospital at midnight. Brent and I pick up my mother for the second time, only this time we believe it's a sure thing. My dad is coming later in the morning. As fate (or God) would have it, Jason's Dad is coming that night to visit for a week. He and his wife have planned a romantic reunion. Instead, Jason and his parents spend the night pacing the floors of the hospital waiting for the pancreas to arrive from California. My heart goes out to them. They all have given selflessly for my benefit. I also feel excitement for Jason. This is something he feels destined to do and the time has arrived!

As I wade through the hours of waiting for the pancreas to arrive, I become less confident. Even though I've had surgery many times, I'm terrified that something will go wrong during the operation. I want to be calm. I want to trust, but the longer I wait, the more I want to run away.

It's now nearly noon, **June 21st**. We've been at the hospital since midnight. The pancreas missed the first flights out of California. I have twenty-four hours from the time it was procured before it can no longer be used. The clock is ticking. I have until 2 P.M. or I will lose the pancreas. The message comes that the pancreas is in a taxi. I think, *A taxi? Really? Some cab driver is carrying my organ in a box in his well-worn back seat?*

At no point did anyone tell me that my risk of surgery was so great that the doctors were uncertain about my survival, but when the doctor in training came in to explain the risks and benefits of the operation to me, he painted an ominous picture. "You're between a rock and a hard place," he said. "We hope you make it." His careless words slap against me. I feel as though I've just been in an explosion. Abject terror rushes through me. I'd had extreme reservations about this whole deal. I've seen the surgeons over and over to be sure I'm making the right decision. I've always known I'm too sick for this colossal operation. The surgeon's words fill me with chilling doom. "I'm not going to do it. Call it off," I say. I whip off the blankets of the bed and I'm sobbing in fear and can't compose myself.

Brent comes quietly to my side and I frantically clutch his hands. I stare into the darkness trying to see into his face. Ever so gently he puts his mouth to my ear, lightly rubbing my cheek with his. He speaks slowly and calmly. "You're going to be fine. You can do this, baby. I'm right here beside you. Listen to me; focus on my voice," he encourages me.

With the help of Brent's eternally calming and loving presence, I am able to gain some composure. I'm still terrified, but I'm willing to go on with the operation.

I'm wheeled into the pre-op holding room. My parents, Brent and my healer are all with me. Each of them has a hand on me and although I'm comforted by their touch, I'm still panic-stricken. Unable to contain my fear any longer, I wail. Dad is holding Mom, who's now also sobbing seeing me so desperate. Hearing the ruckus, the chief surgeon comes to my side. He assuredly strokes my arm and says, "You are going to make it, Shelli, I have no doubt. You will be fine. We aren't a bit worried about you." Although I can still feel my fear, I have to move away from the hysteria I'm feeling and get a grip on myself. I have to focus on trusting that I'm valuable enough to salvage.

In preparation for this moment, I'd posted my thoughts on *my Caring Bridge Journal:*

"...What we're attempting to do here is unnatural, almost sci-fi. This idea of transferring a mass of living cells from a dying person and simultaneously lifting out a living, breathing organ from a second person in order to provide life for a third is something that would have been considered witchcraft in the not so distant past.

"This method of life and surgery that we employ today, I suspect will, indeed, be viewed as barbaric and stone age in the not so distant future. Nonetheless, I am about to attempt something that will, one way or another, forever alter the course of my life.

"I plunge into the deep abyss of the unknown head first, taking in a full, deep breath of myself in order to sustain me in this journey to the other side of my present universe. And like the deep, black velvet void of the un-manifest into which I dive, I become endless and eternal. I have no idea what awaits me. I do know, however, that infinite possibilities are teeming there, in this space of a-morphic, no-thing-ness.

"I have no travel map; no provisions of any sort; no journey companion; no luxury of having done it a hundred times before.

"In my aloneness, though, I know and feel the presence of beings who have always watched over me, who have heard my cries in the night, and have always answered me. I reach up and out to pull these beings close to my questioning and uncertain, fearful thoughts. I begin to have yet another conversation with them, or me, or Him. And like always, the answers come in an easy, uncensored rush.

"I keep with me the one single thing that I cling to, much like a reed embeds itself into the muddy lake's bottom: my utter faith that I am held in love. Held in the love that moves the sun and the stars, as Dante tells us. Held by the love that streaks purple and red and orange in the morning sky. Held by the love that awakens the earth in springtime and lays it to sleep at autumn's end.

"I am a part of all of this. I am not an observer looking in at this majesty, but rather equal to, one of, and aligned with this awesome beauty, love-wisdom. Aligned with the miracle of creation.

"I must believe in such a wondrous entity, whatever its name. If not, what else have I? What else has any of us?

"And so I ask, 'Am I not also miraculous?'

"'Christ in you. The hope of Glory.' Colossians 1:26–27

"And so it is."

-Shelli

When have you stood alone, feeling naked, terrified, and insecure? A double organ transplant isn't commonplace, but feeling as though we are navigating unfamiliar terrain is something everyone can relate to. Even something as natural as becoming a parent is intimidating. We find comfort in familiarity. We like order and predictability--they give us a sense of trust and safety. But if we stay stuck in the known, we miss the opportunity to stretch and evolve. We will never know what greatness we are capable of if we avoid taking risks.

The impulse to grow is an inborn drive. We've been doing it since our conception. This organic desire to continuously evolve never stops. Our souls are just as eager for new experiences when we're fifty-five and seventy-five as when we were five. We can, however, inhibit our growth by succumbing to our insecurities. If we do, eventually our zest for life is dulled. Is there something you've always longed to do, but your apprehension holds you back? Are you waiting for a companion to help you begin a journey that could or should be done alone?

Change is difficult, even if the change is something we've planned for and desire. When we embark on anything new we feel both apprehension and anticipation. When have you made a substantive change in life and felt this? Maybe you've decided to change homes or careers. Maybe you've changed your mind about the nature of a relationship. Or perhaps you've chosen to change the role you were given, and accepted, in your family or society.

As we change and heal our stories, we can feel sadness and remorse, because what we are leaving behind is a part of us. We are leaving the safety and familiarity of what has come to be "normal." We can feel regret for having let so much time go by before being able to produce the courage needed to heal. We feel sad that the old way of seeing our stories doesn't work anymore.

When we're afraid of change and the unknown, our faith can comfort us. We are blessed if we have a person to support us when we're afraid. Most of the time, we have to find our strength from within. This is when we need to have faith in the healing process. We must have faith in something larger than ourselves. We must believe that we are eternally held by and are a part of a kind and loving benevolence.

What is it that sustains you during times of challenge? Beyond our valuable family or friends and our community, we need to be able to anchor ourselves to something that is ever-present. People are important, but they are also limited. Their own emergencies or impulsive desires may inhibit their ability to always respond or to hold us with solidity. I've learned that many of my most desperate times come when the sun isn't up. My irrationality or insistent insecurity can override a warm bath or my doctor's experience. As much as we need the presence and encouraging words of our loved ones, when it comes right down to it, our recycling thoughts can erase our solace with little effort. Find something more stable than the fluctuating nature of the physical to believe in. Even a single tree in the middle of the desolate plains relies on something greater than itself. Surely we, as complicated spiritual and physical beings, need and deserve at least as much as the tree.

PART II

My new kidney worked immediately. My lab values changed overnight and were totally normal! Instead of the expected three-week stay, I was able to go home in six days. I knew I'd been blessed by Jason's sacrifice and by the gift from my pancreas donor, who I call "The Sweet One." All the turmoil and tension of waiting was worth it. I'm euphoric. Leaving the hospital, I'm filled with immeasurable gratitude.

Although I left the hospital with healthy, working organs, the recovery from the double organ transplant took an entire year. It was not at all smooth. I soon learned that transplanting a kidney is the easy part. Pancreas transplants are entirely different. They are finicky and don't like to be moved around. Each day presented something different. I fought off infections and nausea. I was so weak I literally crawled on my hands and knees from room to room, dragging my urine bag and catheter behind me. But my spirit is determined; my warrior of just-causes was called up, and each day I worked at rehabilitation. I progressed slowly until one month following surgery when I experienced a serious complication: severe pancreatitis, an infection in my new pancreas.

I was back in the hospital, critically ill. As a nurse, I already knew what I was up against. Sometimes knowledge is helpful, but this time, I knew too much.

I was delirious and withering from the fevers, vomiting and infection. I was given IV pain medicine that didn't seem to do a thing to comfort me. With the transplant surgery, I'd been given extremely potent immune suppressants to prevent my body from rejecting the new organs. Now those same drugs were preventing my body from fighting the infection. The infection grew and spread to my blood, a condition called, "sepsis." The medical staff was gravely concerned that I would lose my pancreas, or worse, die.

Nights and days ran together. I was shaking with painful rigors and chills, yet my fever continued to soar. I was packed with ice bags, which was torturous. My labs weren't improving. The infection worsened. Antibiotics were increased. I prayed whenever I was coherent. A group of healers prayed for me. What shreds of energy I had I used to focus on faith and positivity. My warrior stood close by. Despite the odds, I was going to survive this and keep my new pancreas!

After more than ten days, medicine and miracles prevail. My body somehow conquered the infection and my pancreas was salvaged.

Even after overcoming that crisis, my unstable medical status required home health care for over three months. A nurse instructed my family about how to give me daily intravenous fluids to keep my blood pressure up. I had blood transfusions to treat low blood counts caused by the immune suppression drugs. The daily challenges and difficulties took all my effort and my family's as well. But the trade-off was that my body had organs that functioned normally! One day, I wrote in my Caring Bridge Journal, "I wish I had a million words to describe how it is that I feel, but all that comes to mind is my hand resting over my abdomen, my new organs working beneath them, and that leaves me speechless."

The whole first year of recovery required my resilience, fortitude, and resolve. I experienced bone marrow suppression, giving cause for alarm because of the possibility of blood cancers. As a result of the dramatic immune suppression, I developed several exquisitely painful lesions under my skin that ate away at the tissue, leaving it necrotic. I underwent surgeries to cut away this dead tissue and was left with large, gaping wounds that required dressing changes twice a day and took weeks to heal. I don't remember how many times during the first year I was required to reach deep into my strength in order to face each day with optimism instead of collapsing into exhausted despair. One time I wrote, "We don't know how much strength we possess until we are called to be strong." Although some days I could only manage to sleep and walk short distances, other days were filled with a progress that inspired me even while encountering these impediments to my recovery.

I'm back at home for three days, the life-threatening pancreatitis and sepsis behind me. I'm resting in a recliner on the sun porch. Looking out the front windows, Brent says, "Hey, your parents are here."

"Dad must have been bored," I say, laughing. Then I get a feeling in my gut I don't like.

My parents come in and we visit. Although they are light-hearted and smiling, happy to see me looking better since the recent hospitalization, I sense something is wrong. I can feel it in my body. In due time Mom takes a deep breath, turns to look at me and says, "I have to tell you that I had a breast biopsy and it came back positive. I have breast cancer."

Deafening silence. My chest heaves with the impact of the news. My lips, hands, and feet tingle as my body goes into shock. I want to roll up her words and stuff them back into her mouth. I put up my hand, "Stop. Stop talking," I say. I believe I'm in a nightmare. I can handle being ill. I'm used to it and know how to overcome it. But not my mother, please, not my mother. I want to get up and run from the room, far away from her words and the unfathomable diagnosis that I find more threatening than anything I've had to endure.

Can anything go smoothly? Must my life be constantly filled with emotional challenges one on top of another? Now I have to not only find faith for my own resurrection, but also for the promise that my mother will be alive and well to remain my steadfast companion. My life filled with medical challenges has tightened our interdependence and connection. I cannot imagine my life without her. I'm terrified, but also angry that I couldn't be granted just one slim moment of peaceful ease and grace.

Mom's own grit emerged as she went through the cancer treatment. She sailed through the lumpectomy and radiation treatments. My own spirit of determination was renewed as I observed her calm confidence. I found the energy to go to the hospital to do energy healing work on her after her surgery in late August. We smiled at one another as I worked on her. What a pair we made! Grinning at me through her grogginess she said to me, "Look at you, Shelli, there you are working away on me with that IV tube dangling from your arm." And life went on.

Each day my new organs worked like they had always belonged to me. I was awestruck at how I experienced life differently without diabetes and kidney failure dictating how I felt. Gone were the hourly battles of attempting to maintain a normal blood sugar level. No longer did I live with the threat of falling into a coma without warning. The need for Brent to give me IV insulin while standing in our kitchen evaporated! I had the peace of mind that my new kidney was safe from the ravages of the ugly, sinister disease that had already stolen so much of my vitality, stolen so much of my life. My experience of being alive morphed into bliss.

All those years of crying on the bathroom floor, beseeching God for my salvation. Now it had arrived. With a healthy kidney, the threat of dialysis was over. All the chemistries of my body were normal. I felt physically robust. With my healthy kidney and no diabetes, my weight fell by nearly 50 pounds. I was beginning to believe that the sweetness and ease of life I had lost so many decades ago was within my grasp.

One day in October Brent and I went to dinner with his brother and wife. Instead of scrutinizing the menu for something I could eat that was within my renal and diabetic diets, I ordered whatever I wanted: a carbohydrate-laden meal of squash ravioli with caramelized onions, ginger ale, and bread pudding for dessert. Dessert, I'm ordering dessert! I savored every morsel. After the meal we walked to our car. Settling into my seat I began an automatic analysis of how I felt inside. Something was off. To my amazement, I felt nothing, at least that's what I thought. I said to Brent, "This is about the time I'd start to feel like shit. But I don't." I was overcome by my awareness that my body worked like it was supposed to!

In that moment, I realized the thirty-five–year war with diabetes was over.

By June of the following year, I was experiencing fewer side effects from the medications. I had not been in the hospital for a few months and I felt terrific every day. In celebration, Brent and I hosted a gala, a one–year post–surgery party at our home. Jason's parents flew back to attend. He was the hero of the party! My friends and family brought him gifts and we all thanked him for his selflessness and for saving my life. Truly he was, and is, the hero in the story. Without his kidney, I'd still be sick and I wouldn't have been able to receive the pancreas. My friends and family were thrilled to see how great Jason was doing after his operation. He had met a woman and was in love, planning their long-term life together.

My new organs functioned with spot–on accuracy until almost two years after the transplant. Between my lab tests in February and March of 2010, my monthly blood test numbers suddenly changed dramatically. The pancreas was once again in serious trouble. I was rattled with fear. If I rejected the pancreas, I would return to the life that nearly destroyed me. The only accurate way to tell if rejection is present is by doing a biopsy of the organ. This is generally a simple test. Few things are simple for me, however.

I go into the hospital **for** the biopsy. The plan is for the interventional radiologist to insert a long needle through my abdomen and into the pancreas. She will take three small samples of pancreas tissue to examine. There will be changes in the tissue if the organ is rejecting. The physician has difficulty finding an area where the pancreas isn't covered by loops of intestines. If she punctures the intestine, I could become seriously or fatally ill. After much maneuvering a good spot is located and the tissue samples are obtained.

The doctor examines the tissue under a microscope in the procedure room. I lie on the table as she studies each sample. I hear words that can't possibly be true: "Your pancreas is dead," the doctor blurts out. The heavy sedation I've been given dulls my perceptions and emotions, but her words come through uncensored. "Dead? What do you mean, dead?" I slur. I'm in a state of disbelief. The doctor's voice shouts through the fog of the sedation, "There is nothing here but fibrous tissue. The organ has moved into deep rejection. This is what we see when the organ tissue dies."

I'm destroyed. I'm wheeled back to my outpatient room to recover. I lay numb. *It's gone. I'm back to diabetes. It will start to kill my new kidney.* I feel dazed, yet simultaneously unspeakably grief–stricken. I'm so despondent that even tears are impossible. Nurses I know come to see me, but I lay silent and immobile in my misery.

The biopsy tissue is sent to pathology for further analysis. This report will be back in a couple of days. Back at home, Brent and I once again look at one another in a long moment of silence. He says, "I don't believe it's true."

I say, "Neither do I, but it's hard to deny what she said."

Brent says, "I'm not going to buy this until the biopsy comes back from the pathologist."

We wait. I vacillate between my fear and my faith. I hear the voices that want to drag me into the depths of doubt and my old ways of thinking that God is out to get me. When I hear these voices that want to rekindle my suspicion and mistrust, I intentionally turn my focus to faith and my belief in a God whose love is limitless. I am immersed in that source of beauty.

Making this choice mandates conscious effort. I deliberately chase away the diagnosis the doctor gave me in the procedure room. Instead, I repeat the mantra that I am held by a love so unconditional nothing can penetrate its protection. I hold fiercely to my faith. My belief fortifies my hope. If I lose hope, I've lost everything.

I'm trying to relax by getting a facial. I'm lying on the lounge; the esthetician I've known for years is massaging oils into my face. My cell phone rings. It's the University. They have my pathology report. "We want to let you know that all of the tissue we got was muscle, no pancreas tissue. We don't know the condition of your pancreas, but the fibrous tissue was your muscle." I leap from the lounge! Judy and I jump and hug and dance. "Thank you, thank you, God," we both shout.

"I knew it had to be wrong!" I say. I'm spirited into an even stronger resolve to continue to hold the hand of hope despite my circumstance.

Since the biopsy was a failure, another test was ordered to be sure the pancreas was getting adequate blood. The test showed the blood flow was normal, so that isn't the cause of the poor lab results. It's looking more and more probable that I'm rejecting the pancreas. But the test revealed another more menacing issue: a mass on my native kidney and adrenal gland that is highly suspicious for cancer.

How much more can I take? Now I'm facing pancreas rejection and I need to contend with the possibility that I have cancer. If someone tried to make my life into a movie, no one would believe it!

I feel utterly exhausted, sad, terrified. I feel as though I'm being shot at from all directions with no safe haven. *What the hell! How many times am I going to be trampled? How many times must I pick myself up? How much can one person take?*

I feel as though everything I've strived for over the past two years is unraveling before me and I'm impotent to stop it. I'm compelled to do something, anything, to take some sort of positive action. Since I know how powerful words are, I decide I have to claim these organs as my own. Saturated with fear and desperation I hastily write an entry in my Caring Bridge Journal. I mention that my kidney is doing fine. I go on to say that I'm calling it "my" kidney now, and I won't be calling it "Jason's kidney" anymore, because it's not. Though my intention was that this affirmation would bring more solidity to the organs, the statement ended up being a mistake I regret.

The only way to tell if the mass on my native kidney and adrenal gland is cancerous or not was by surgically removing both structures and performing a biopsy. Since the surgeon was already inside my abdomen doing this procedure, he was now able to take a clean sample of the pancreas to test for rejection as well. As I was admitted for the operation I realize that this will be my sixth operation in less than two years. The surgery may prove I have cancer and that I'm rejecting my pancreas.

The operation is called a "total radical nephrectomy" and it is radical! A good deal of tissue is torn inside during the operation. For many weeks following the surgery, I had uncontrollable, burning pain. In the midst of this, I'm distraught about an e-mail I receive from Jason.

Jason read my posting that I would be calling the new kidney "mine" now and that it was no longer his kidney. He was very hurt. He wrote me saying that he felt I got what I wanted, his kidney, and then "kicked him to the curb." He said he thought I ought to show some gratitude, and that it would be better if we never spoke again. I felt as though I was run over by a tank. I was sick to think he would actually feel these thoughts and emotions about me. I could understand his being upset and needing to say so, but to go so far as to say I was ungrateful and to cut off all ties felt extreme.

Once home recovering from the kidney removal, my nurse at the university called with the pathology report on the tumor. "I'm sorry to tell you that it's cancer, Shelli. You need to make an appointment with an oncologist." The weight of his words lay on me with such pressure I'm unable to continue standing. I sink into a chair. I call my parents. Mom answers. "It's cancer," I say. Her voice is grief-stricken, "Oh, Shelli." I say, "I'm sorry, *Mom, I'm so sorry.*" Silent tears burn my cheeks. What now?

I am also, indeed, in pancreatic rejection. I'm crawling, struggling to hold on to any shadow of hope and faith. It all feels like way too much for one human being to handle. I cry for hours. I lay on my treatment table of my meditation room, seeking solace and courage. The next day I once again reach into the deep place inside me and get ready to rise above the oppressive news. I'm ready to fight for my right to live.

I'm unable to take the full treatment for the organ rejection because of the new cancer diagnosis. The treatment for the pancreas rejection is to give me drugs that gravely suppress my immune system so that the pancreas feels less like a foreign entity to my body. If the doctors give me the full immune-suppressing treatment, it can cause the cancer to spread. I feel like a rabbit stuck in the middle of a highway. It seems any direction I turn is already pre-set for disaster.

In the midst of this heartbreaking medical news, I can't get Jason out of my mind. My relationship with him is important to me. I'm tormented day and night about how to handle Jason's feelings. Re-reading my post, I can understand how my words could have been misunderstood. I updated my Caring Bridge Journal to explain what I hadn't taken the time to put into words earlier. I thought people would understand that I was terrified and trying everything I could to keep all my donated parts alive. The fact that Jason donated a part of his body for my benefit was never lost to me, but I believe he took it that way. I anguished over Jason's dismissal for many weeks as I underwent the treatment for the pancreas rejection and recovered from having my cancerous, native kidney removed.

I was finally graced with some positive news: The type of cancer I had in my kidney was curable with surgery. It was detected early and hadn't spread to any other structures or the lymph system. I felt as though the mild pancreas rejection was a necessary event that detected the cancer at an early stage. Sometimes not getting what you want is a stroke of luck.

A client of mine offered to organize a healing circle at our home and I enthusiastically accepted. The healing circle took place on the back patio at our home. Many people attended to pray, offering positive affirmations, and to simply sit with the visualization of my lab values returning to baseline. We had a specific number on which to focus. Within two weeks, I had returned to my pre-rejection number. My surgeon was astonished since I had only been given a partial treatment for the rejection. This coupled with the news that I had a cancer that was considered cured ignited and renewed my faith and belief in infinite possibilities.

I extended an olive branch to Jason and gratefully, he took it. We talked on the phone. I felt comforted that Jason came to feel no regret about a decision that was so monumental for both of us, and happy that he and I were a team again. Hopefully, all would go smoothly from here on out, but not so.

It's now been four years since the double organ transplant. I'm teaching class at Rukha, the school of healing that Brent and I operate, when I feel a tremendous pain in my abdomen. After class that evening, I go to the emergency department. My labs show that my kidney is failing. I'm admitted to the hospital. Many tests are done to determine the reason why my kidney would fail so long after transplant. The tests come up empty. Doctors are baffled. Each day my kidney function declines. The situation is quite grave. Surprisingly, I'm worried, but not panicked. As

I talk with Brent, I use my intuitive abilities to investigate what could be wrong. "There's something impeding the blood flow," I say to Brent and the doctors. But the tests show blood flow to be normal. The doctors are puzzled and they're willing to take my intuition into consideration. They order more scans of my kidney. Something interesting shows up in these sequential scans: my kidney is spinning like a top in my abdomen! When it spins, the artery is choked off. Then it unwinds, usually because I'm running my hands over it to detect what's wrong and to give it energy. This winding and unwinding has released the strangulation of the artery and prevented the kidney from dying!

I have yet another operation to secure my kidney to the back of my abdominal muscle. In the history of kidney transplant, I'm the 17th person in the world to have this occur.

The story of the kidney–pancreas never ends. Being an organ recipient, there is no finish line, no moment when I can rest knowing my body will work effectively, without complications caused by the immune suppressing medications that keep the organs functioning. I'm grateful for the opportunity organ transplant has given me to continue my life, which is a very good life.

When I was gifted Scott's kidney when I was twenty-five years old, my life was extended by twenty-one years. I realized many dreams during that time. Since then, I've had a full and rich life that has been blessed. With the gift of Jason's kidney and the pancreas from The Sweet One, for the first time in my adult life my physical body has been able to keep up with my spiritual body. This blessing allows me to do the work I believe I came to do: healing myself and helping others to experience their own magnificence through the healing found in their own stories.

Six years after this operation, I was again faced with an even greater challenge, one that put to the test all the emotional and spiritual healing I'd thus far accomplished.

THE HEALING

Through the story of my double organ transplant, I learned lessons about receptivity, the ease that harmony allows, and the immeasurable pleasure and power of gratitude.

I'm often overcome with awe and wonder at what my body has, and is, able to endure. I feel reverent gratitude for these organs that have managed to integrate and ultimately, become me, even though they weren't part of my original system. It strikes me how the kidney and pancreas have internal wisdom. I witnessed how they have such implacable self-awareness, that even though their environment was changed, they still held tight to their identity in *my* body. Although the pancreas struggled, she settled into the universe of my body willingly, like the kidney.

As I waited through the weeks and months for the pancreas offer, I reflected on the enormity of what I was asking my body to do: take on two more outside organs. I started seeing the organs as entire planets leaving their original solar system and moving into mine. When I had my first kidney transplant, I was very young and thought of the organ exchange in a simplified way. Now I have evolved and have a more sophisticated comprehension of the energy and the consciousness of living things.

I realized that in order for the organ exchange to work, harmony needed to be present. I felt awed that two organs could simply adapt and live harmoniously in my body with a little support from medications.

Experiencing this beautiful interface and acceptance helped me recognize how often I, as a human being, don't have the same tolerance for people, cultures, and beliefs that are foreign to me. I've never considered myself a bigot. But the surgery made me honestly look at the parts of me that held bigoted, righteous thoughts and judgments, and to diligently work to consciously change them. I've healed a lot of them, but I know if I were to be totally transparent, I can find judgments and beliefs in me that don't promote a harmonious interface among all peoples. My newfound awareness helps me to stay attentive to any exclusionary ideas in my belief system. I'm grateful to have the opportunity to be witness to my thoughts that go against my value of equality.

Jason had made a significant sacrifice; the event was life-changing for both of us. I said to him, "I would hate to think that you would regret an act that was so tremendous, so meaningful." I'll never again underestimate the healing power of validating someone's experience, whether or not it matches my own.

In receiving the pancreas from the seventeen-year old girl from California, I struggled with my worthiness in being the one who got to live. Receptivity had always been difficult for me. I'm much more comfortable giving to others than receiving, probably because receiving requires a fair amount of vulnerability. Receiving requires me to accept and admit that I have needs. I couldn't imagine a more intense way to learn that lesson than to have a viable person die in order that I might live.

I made peace with the fact that I have needs and that's okay so long as they are appropriate. I realized the difference between my "special needs" as someone who has multiple disabilities and the distortion of being "needy." I found myself dependent on the mercy of others, whether they were my organ donors, those who helped me recover for months following the surgery, or the dedicated nurses and physicians. Being dependent helped me to heal the fallacy I had about my legitimate needs being "too much" and thus, labeling myself "a pain in the ass." Although I was often terrified of the vulnerability I felt having to rely on others, I also learned that this type of dependency didn't mean I was a slacker or a weak person.

I have enormous gratitude for Jason and his family, for the family of my pancreas donor, for my own family and friends, and for the hard work of the extremely skilled surgeons and nurses. Without each of them, I would simply not be alive today. I feel incredibly humbled and healed. My gratitude is an emotion, a tangible sensation running through my body, through my heart, that I haven't previously known. The words seem small, but there's so much meaning behind them when I say "thank you." The entire experience not only saved my life, but changed it in ways I did not anticipate and could not have imagined.

Needs are a struggle for everyone. Some of us deny our needs and never ask for help, even when it is warranted. Others ask for help when they are, or ought to be, perfectly capable of managing for themselves. The healing task is to find balance between these two extremes, and accept help graciously and gratefully, and realize our capabilities and accept responsibility for our independence. If you're on a journey of healing, here are some steps to begin gaining awareness about your needs: Take a look at your behaviors in relation to your needs. Are they too independent or not independent enough? Are you accepting of help or do you refuse and insist on doing everything on your own (and then are resentful because no one is helping you)? Do you feel that people ought to know what you need without asking, and if you have to ask for what you need, do you feel unloved or unseen?

You probably haven't had a double organ transplant or kidney cancer, but it's likely you've had to rely on the charity and goodness of others at some time in your life. Needing help can feel scary because it makes us feel dependent and vulnerable. What is your reaction when you feel exposed and at the mercy of others? If you collapse when you feel vulnerable, or conversely, if you deny your fear and become fierce and cocky, you have some healing to do related to vulnerability. In the middle ground between these two polarized positions, there is a sweet spot where we're not afraid of our vulnerability. Amazingly, we even appreciate it.

Being able to appreciate the power of our vulnerability first requires that we become aware of our limiting beliefs about how we view people who need help. Do you believe as I used to that autonomy and self-reliance are the "better" qualities over humility and sensitivity? Being independent isn't bad, but we need to find balance in our independence so that we are self-reliant and accepting of our limitations.

Learning humility and the art of seeing situations from another's viewpoint requires us to ignore our ego's need to be right, and instead, respond to our soul's desire for harmony. The ego believes it is right and feels threatened by any attempt to silence it. Have you jeopardized important relationships because you can't let go of your ego's righteousness? Before we can learn to stand in the shoes of another, it is necessary to recognize our own judgmental thoughts, biases, and bigotry. Openly admitting to these parts of ourselves is threatening. We believe that good people don't have bad thoughts. The truth is, we all have prejudice, bigotry, and righteousness that we learned early on in our story. The cultures in which we live teach us our biases. Our families, religious dogma, social constructs, and real life experiences color our perceptions. Looking at life from this polarized perspective is useful at first; it helps us differentiate ourselves from others. Knowing our individual identity is an important milestone in our psychological development. As we mature, however, this narrow cone of perception becomes limiting and is no longer useful.

Once we realize that we've been conditioned to think in a prejudiced, self-absorbed way, it's easier to admit the truth of our thoughts. And once we admit them, they are no longer lurking in shadow. Our admission moves us from pretense toward authenticity.

If we wish to live as the radiant, glorious beings of love that God hopes us to be, we become motivated to widen our perspective and modify our exclusive beliefs that set us apart and above others. We become naturally motivated to heal attitudes that create divisiveness and the artificial hierarchy that maintains exclusivity.

Until we're willing to heal this split from our true nature, we will always harbor anger and hostility. These will always create a sense of lack in our lives: lack of compassion, lack of forgiveness, lack of happiness, lack of worth and respect both for others and for ourselves. Are you able to see how your heritage, where you live, and your real-life experiences have set you up to have exclusionary beliefs and opinions? Are you willing to become transparent and acknowledge these judgments and prejudices? If so, list them to see where your healing work begins in this area. Be concise. Do you root for the underdog, but judge people who are successful? Do you believe the only way to piety is through minimalism? Can people who drive luxury cars and who dress in designer clothing also be good and humble? Do you value the arts and judge those who love professional sports or game shows? Do you believe all Western medicine is poison, the hospitals villainous? Or conversely, do you believe homeopathic or spiritual interventions to health are fads, the practitioners quacks? Practice having an opinion rather than a judgment. Examine how your heritage, value system or other factors influence your biases and tendencies to label and to judge.

As we heal our early conditioning, we are able to leave behind the dualistic model that says we are either a success or a failure, and instead, realize that all thoughts and characteristics are honorable in so much as our greed can awaken us to our generosity, our intolerance directs us toward our acceptance, and our boastfulness is a signal to invite our humility. This new consciousness enables us to accept and internalize the truth that we, along with all people, all cultures and all groups, regardless of socio-economic status, ability or disability, color or creed, are born of the same Divinity and thus, are inherently deserving of respect and compassion.

We don't change spontaneously. Instead, our growth emerges gradually through consistent attention to our process of internal healing. When we heal our ego-based instincts that hold us separate from others, we are automatically inclined toward graciousness and reverence for the whole of humanity, which includes the self.

With persistence you can learn to embrace your legitimate needs and feel your worth. You can temper your righteous ego that urges you to defend your position and instead, become open to hear another's voice and the truth of their experience. Healing the distortions of your stories will create desire for harmony in your life. It will show you that comparing and competing creates tension and anxiety. When you view all of humanity as equal, you will be naturally inclined to respond to the opportunity to give selflessly to others, not for praise or for fame, but for the love of humanity and to be of service. When you expand your consciousness to this level, you will feel an ecstatic ripple of gratitude flood your heart, and you will find miracles in the ordinary.

"Even if it's a little thing, do something for others -
something for which you get no pay
but the privilege of doing it."
Albert Schweitzer

"If you don't know what you want, you'll never find it. If you
don't know what you deserve, you'll always settle for less.
You will wander aimlessly, uncomfortably numb in your
comfort zone, wondering how life has ended up here."
Rob Liano

"You are only afraid if you are not in harmony with yourself.
People are afraid because they have never
owned up to themselves."
Herman Hesse

Chapter Eight

OUR LIVING SOULS

APRIL 2014

I'M AT HOME GETTING READY FOR WORK WHEN MY PHONE RINGS. GOING to the kitchen, I answer it. It's a nurse from the oncologist's office. She has the results of a CT scan of my neck and chest that was done the previous day. The weekend before I'd been working with a client when I casually scratched my collarbone. My fingers landed on a node no bigger than a sesame seed. I knew it shouldn't be there. I called my oncologist who then scheduled a CT scan.

Standing calmly in my work clothes, prepared for an ordinary day, I listen to the nurse. "The doctor would like to see you this morning to discuss your scan, Shelli." Being a nurse for the past thirty years, I know doctors don't call the day after a CT scan asking you to come to the office that very day if the scan is normal. I also know she's holding the report in her hand. "What does the report say?" I ask.

As I listen to her response, my here–and–now evaporates. I enter a timeless place. I drift untethered, no longer connected to anything. I'm gone, but I don't know where. "You have a single enlarged node at your neck and multiple diffuse tumors throughout your back and sternum. You also have three nodules in the left lower lobe of your lung and two in your right lung." I'm listening, knowing my life will never be the same. The nurse goes on to say words that again, cannot be true: "It appears that you have metastatic small cell lung cancer, Shelli."

A surge of something I've never felt before travels through my body. I feel as though my bones and flesh have turned to liquid. I continue to stand while I hold the phone to my ear; my other hand on the black and white granite island, keeps me from falling over. I'm a transplant patient. I absolutely will not survive metastatic small cell lung cancer. I have six months tops.

I hang up the phone. I stand unmoving in the kitchen listening for what I should do next. I have no idea how to feel what I heard. My hand runs over the cool granite; from the living room I hear the grandfather clock steadily tick. I'm going to die this year. Hearing the unwavering tick of the clock I realize that I cannot stop time nor make it go backward. In the living room, time proceeds onward. But my time will soon end.

As I re-connect to the present moment, a thought gently enters: *So this is how it will end; my life journey is over.* A most unfamiliar sense of peace overtakes me. While I'm impacted by the nurse's information, I'm neither devastated nor overwhelmed with fear. I'm not wishing to run from the news like I have wanted to do at other times. One of my first thoughts is that I will finally be released from my interminable prison of darkness, and the isolation and intolerable limitations I so often feel trapped within. But another voice clearly speaks behind these thoughts: *Do not believe this; it isn't true.* The peace I feel is not abiding.

I'm not at all expecting to be diagnosed with a fatal illness. The double organ transplant six years ago radically changed my life experience. Free from kidney disease and diabetes, Brent and I are less hyper-vigilant about possible health disasters.

I feel vibrant most every day! We are enjoying life more fully: traveling, hiking, eating out with friends, going to concerts, and remodeling our home. I literally feel reborn and do everything I can to maintain my health and keep my new organs happy. I eat a mostly organic diet. I'm vehement about my daily exercise and I maintain an even more ardent spiritual practice. The renal cell cancer that was found four years ago is barely a memory in my mind. With my new-found energy, I've opened a licensed school of energy medicine in Minnesota and have increased my sessions with my private clients in my professional healing practice. I faithfully have my blood work done every month. By all accounts, I'm extremely healthy.

Back in my kitchen, in the real moment, I realize I have to tell Brent what I was told. I walk on legs that feel boneless, down the stairs to the bathroom where Brent is shaving, getting ready for his ordinary day. I stand in the doorway. "I have lung cancer," I report to him in a tone that's matter-of-fact, my face absent of emotion. I'm unable to feel, to think. I'm not even sure I'm still breathing. Standing there, my skin tingles and in the recesses of my mind, the words I'm speaking float indifferently in the air.

"What?" Brent says in disbelief as he steps toward me. "How can this be?" he asks, his voice squeezed.

"I don't know. The nurse just called and told me my CT looks as though I have metastatic lung cancer that has spread to my chest and back." The sense of composure I had in the kitchen dies. The nurse's words register in my mind. Silent tears slide down my cheeks. Brent comes to me and grips me fiercely. We stand in the bathroom silently crying together. What's the sense of words?

Brent abruptly lets go and pushes me aside, "I can't take this." He rushes from the bathroom. I let him alone to process the news that his wife who lifts weights, hikes on wooded trails every week, works vibrantly at three jobs she loves, and drinks organic vegetable shakes for breakfast, will soon be eaten away by lung cancer.

We drive to the hospital where we both work. We have two hours to endure before the appointment with the oncologist in the next building. I'm reminded of a healer who I worked with some years ago. He works with cancer patients. Desperate for help of any kind, I dial his cell phone, which I've not called in years, and miraculously, he answers! I explain the situation. He says to me, "Well, let's change the report." We hang up and he does whatever he does. I don't care what he does as long as it erases what I was told standing in my kitchen.

Brent and I arrive at the oncologist's office. I'm so tense with fear that I'm not sure I'll hear anything I'm told. I ask my friend, a cancer certified nurse who works in the hospital with me, to come with us.

The doctor reviews the same information the nurse gave me on the phone about the tumors. He tells me the next step is to have the node surgically removed and a biopsy done. He says, "At this point we have no idea what it is; it could be an infection." I'm clenching Brent's hand so tightly I can't feel my fingers. Listening to the oncologist, I begin to cry. *Why is he telling me they don't know what it is when the nurse already told me that the report said it was lung cancer?* I'm too terrified to ask him the question. I look to my friend, who knows what I was told.

My friend looks at the doctor and says, "Shelli got different news from your nurse this morning. Shelli was told that she has lung cancer."

The doctor is obviously surprised. He's adamant as he looks at the report on his computer screen, "No! There is nothing in this report that says anything about lung cancer. We have no idea what this is without a biopsy."

I feel the unfaltering presence of the God I've come to know enfold me as I recall my conversation with the healer an hour ago, *"Let's change the report."*

In the ten days before the biopsy I dance between trust and mistrust, confidence and collapse. All the spiritual healing I've done is put to test. I am aware of the part of me that believes I am unalterably aligned with Universal Goodness and the love of God. I can feel the part of me that will endure whatever lies ahead. I'm also aware of my human side that feels powerless and trampled. I don't even try to pretend I'm purely confident. At this moment I'm tired of lessons and growth and finding healing within the pain. I want reprieve. I'm enlightened enough!

I meditate twice daily. I ask for the love of Jesus as I've done so many times before. My healed self remembers that Source, God, is unconditional love. In a meditation, a giant heart descends toward me from above. As it nears me, it takes on the appearance of a traditional Valentine heart; covered in lace and glowing from inside. It sinks into my chest. As it does, I experience a visceral sensation in my heart center. It's warm, expanding and I'm filled with the sense of a love so great I weep. I dissolve into this love, allowing it to soothe my fears. Stillness abides within me and I remember the previous times this love has carried me.

Nighttime is the worst time for me. My thoughts run wild. The nurse's words haunt me. I wonder what it will be like to die by the end of this year. I shake my head and return to the oncologist's words, "We don't know what this is." I remember the healer's words, "Let's change the report." I'm tormented by the voices battling in my head. I finally find sleep each night when I choose to lean on my steady faith.

The surgeon approaches me after the biopsy. I'm in the recovery room. "The node is malignant, but we don't know what type of cancer it is until we get the pathology back. It will be a week or so." Really? Why not just beat me with a hammer instead? Each hour feels like a year. I've waited too long already and I haven't even heard the diagnosis or started the treatment. I remember a quote of Mother Theresa's: "I know God won't give me more than I can handle; I just wish He didn't trust me so much."

Brent and I return to the oncologist's office for the results of the biopsy. Do I have lung cancer? What is my prognosis? I'm rigid with apprehension. I want him to hurry up and speak, make it fast so it won't hurt so much. Being strong is getting old. I don't want to be brave any more. I'm worn out. I feel as though I've been tossed from shore to sea like a piece of driftwood for decades. I wish I could return to my childhood of sweetness and ease.

The biopsy results show I have "diffuse B-cell lymphoma." The oncologist is almost smiling. Relief pours through my body like rain. I'm being told I have a cancer that's serious, but it is a treatable condition, so long as it has not spread to my bone marrow or other organs. I have a good cancer, incredulous as that sounds. This particular type of cancer has been well studied, the exact treatment is known. The lymphoma is a direct result of the immune suppression from the transplant medications, and the transplants are a direct result of the diabetes. Although the diabetes is treated as long as my transplanted pancreas works properly, it is not gone. It is a chronic disease without a cure. It continues to interfere with my longing and ability to live healthfully and with vibrancy. More than blindness, I hate diabetes. Given the chance to be cured of one or the other, I would choose diabetes without a moment's hesitation. Blindness can't kill me, diabetes still can.

I go to work every day, not doing a hell of a lot, but staying home only drives me insane. I'm now having incredible pain day and night. I'm prescribed strong narcotics that make it tolerable to breathe, but not to move. The unrelenting pain is searing through my back and chest. I've developed tumors that are now visible on my chest and abdomen. One is over my collar bone and I fear it's invaded the bone. Even without a scan, we can see the cancer spreading and growing just by looking at me. The rapid changes are daunting and make it difficult to stay positive. I hate knowing that with every passing day, the cancer cells are dividing rapidly and taking over what were once healthy cells. I feel like time is being wasted as we wait for test results. I'm concerned the waiting is giving the cancer time to invade my organs, and it's the truth! My biggest worry is the nodules that were found in my lungs. These can be anything: lymphoma or another type of cancer, including lung cancer. Given my immune suppression, surviving lung cancer is highly improbable.

I need to have a biopsy of the nodules in my lungs to diagnose what they are but that will come later. I need two more tests to stage the cancer: a bone marrow biopsy and a PET scan. A PET scan is a highly sensitive test used to detect even a single cancer cell anywhere in the body. I undergo the bone marrow biopsy as soon as possible and schedule the PET scan for the following week.

The marathon of tests, procedures, and surgeries is like navigating a minefield. Just because I've made it past one test doesn't mean my next step won't result in disaster. Brent and I both agonize over the procedures and wait for a final prognosis. Even though tension is present and real, we set about life with focus each day. We go to work, pray, meditate, hike at the lake and love one another with open honesty each night. We remind one another daily that we are a team and our faith will carry us.

I'm sitting in a tiny **room** by myself in the basement of the hospital. I've been given an injection of radioactive sugar for the PET scan. My mobile phone rings. It's the oncology clinic. I know they are calling with the results of my bone marrow biopsy. There's no way in hell I'm answering that call now. If I hear the cancer is already in my bone marrow, the PET scan is unnecessary; hope for long-term survival will not be possible for me. I let the call go to voice mail.

Back at home, I put off listening to the message for hours; I can't bring myself to hear it. I hold my phone in my hand, running my thumb over the face. Abruptly, I hand the phone to Brent, "I can't do it. You have to listen and then tell me. And if it's bad don't tell me anything," I say, and

I walk across the room to stand far away from the phone.

After listening to the message he announces with an air of conviction, "It's normal."

I laugh and cry at the same time. Brent and I rush to one another with relief and hold tightly in a long embrace. Our journey together has already been so unusual and riddled with life-and-death moments. We know the next phase of our journey won't be smooth, but the past triumphant moments serve as a bedrock for our optimism.

Time drags. Although it's only two days before I can learn the results of the PET scan and meet the oncologist who will treat me, not knowing is excruciating and taxing. Remaining optimistic is much harder without knowing what I'm facing and how much courage and strength I'll be required to find.

Brent and I sit in Dr. Holtan's office, the oncologist who will treat the cancer. She notices my plum colored boots with peace signs and hearts and four-leaf clovers and makes a comment. Her cheerfulness frightens me. I believe she's trying to distract me from the dismal news she has to give. I'm in unspeakable pain. The tumor on my collarbone is protruding through my cheerful yellow sweater. She reviews a number of things. Finally, we get the results we've waited for. "The lymphoma is totally isolated to your lymphatic system," she says.

I feel light headed and I let my held breath go. "Are you sure?" I ask her.

"Yes, I'm sure," she replies.

I simply cannot believe what I'm hearing. I think she must be missing something. What about the nodules in my lungs? I don't want to release my grip on my fear until I triple-confirm the results. I press her over and over again.

"There are no nodules in your lungs, Shelli."

I'm speechless and sit in confused silence. After a bit of time, I say, "The CT showed nodules in the lower lobes of both lungs. You should be able to see them better on the PET scan." Dr. Holtan agrees and reviews both the radiologist's report of the scan and looks at each image herself. I want to look myself, but can't. I urgently direct Brent, "Get up! Get up! I need you to look!" He stands behind her and begins to search the scan with her.

"No, there are no nodules showing up in your lungs."

I wilt into the chair and Brent holds me tightly against him. I weep tears of joy. I've been meditating on the nodules. I've had energy healing work done on them. I've been praying, along with countless others. They are gone! In the span of three weeks I've gone from being told I have metastatic lung cancer with five nodules in my lungs to having them disappear. I'm swept up in the truth that all things are possible! Even for me, an ordinary person.

I have stage III lymphoma. The treatment is already specific and known; I will have six chemotherapy treatments three weeks apart. The treatment is more complex in my case. I have to reduce the immune suppression medications that keep my organs working. It is important that my immune system be bolstered to help the chemotherapy work in treating the tumors. But I need enough immune suppression to prevent my organs from rejecting. Finding the perfect balance that maintains the organs and cures the cancer is a very thin string stretched over what feels like the Grand Canyon.

I've been called to manage this tightrope so many times before. I fully realize what I'm up against with this diagnosis and treatment, and yet I have unflappable belief and confidence, not from arrogance, but from my trust and faith that I am living a Divine plan that doesn't end here.

PART TWO

I believe I've overcome much in my life by making a clear decision to survive. I realize death is much closer than many of us think. Now, I'm even more deliberate in my decision to choose life. So long as I have freedom to choose, I have sovereignty. In sovereignty I can find a reason to live, and that's what I did. When I thought I had lung cancer, I not only realized, but felt just how close death is. Even with the less deadly lymphoma, I understood I was at a crossroad; I could decide the treatment was too difficult, my body and spirit too tired after years of physical hardships. I could focus on how incredibly hard life is some days. Or I could embrace the parts of my life that are abundant and beautiful. I love my life experience, despite it not being perfect. I am happy more days than I'm upset, I know I still have work to do here and I'm not ready for my human experience to end.

I'm not in a state of denial about the seriousness of my condition. Even though I understand that people die from this cancer, I remain faithful in my belief that my time is not up. Thinking back on this belief today, I can see the irony in it. People who don't think it's their time and are diagnosed with a fatal illness die every day. Why am I any different? Perhaps the difference is that I expect miracles as ordinary events rather than occasional mysteries.

Although medical experts use the word "cure" I also know how lethal lymphoma can be for transplant patients. I ought to feel some terror that I have an aggressive, systemic cancer. But I'm experiencing an angel holding me, and I feel a lot of peace. Even before the exact diagnosis was made, I knew I was about to have an experience that would show me I am more than who I thought I was or could ever be. I knew my spirit must remain aligned with God. I knew I had to keep my physical body as strong as possible to endure the treatments. I understood that my attitude needed to reflect my inner faith and positivity. I knew that if I projected an image of confidence, others would gather strength in their faith about my outcome as well. I knew I would need to call on all of my inner and outer resources to come out of this not only alive, but becoming even more of my true self: my soul.

I can't wait to start the cure, as I call it. My best friend, Beth, declared that "C" is for "cure" rather than "cancer." The pain in my back is worse than anything I've experienced. I set my alarm an hour before I need to get up so I can take two pain pills. Without them, merely sitting up in bed is excruciating. Even with the narcotics, I'm only able to be upright for five minutes at a time before I have to lie down again, or lean over on my bathroom vanity, gasping for breath. Although I believe it isn't possible to experience more pain, I feel noticeably worse with each passing day. Brent feels helpless watching me. There's nothing he can do to help, other than to take over every conceivable task, sometimes even putting my shoes on for me. I'm determined, some say willful, and I go to work every day. I lead a four-hour introductory healing workshop. I have to take two pain pills half way through. I push onward because if I'm alone with nothing purposeful to focus on, my resolve shrinks into uncertainty, fear, and doubt. My clarity morphs too easily to confusion.

Today is the Monday after **Easter.** Mom sits with me all day at the hospital waiting for the first chemo treatment to begin. I take IV pain medicine and for the first time in many weeks, the pain is tolerable. We watch old movies and talk about the past and the future. Finally, after waiting all day, I get my first chemo drug at six in the evening. As my young male nurse watches from the side, Mom and I hold the first chemo medication in its double-bagged plastic container in our hands. We begin a ritual I started years ago with medication. We pray our intention into the seemingly benign liquid. "You are filled with the radiance of God; you are assigned the task from Source to lovingly and compassionately enter my body and remove all that does not serve God and leave all other cells undamaged. I am grateful for your immense wisdom in knowing exactly how to do this. Thank you. I love you. Please forgive me. I'm grateful. You are 100% pure love. And so it is."

My nurse, John, is fascinated. "I've never seen anything like that," he remarks in a soft voice filled with wonder.

The liquid in the bag is neither innately good nor bad. It has the ability to receive the consciousness, the "kavanah" –a Hebrew word meaning *intention,* of our hands and our words. The molecules making up the liquid will change, become more brilliant in their geometric pattern, following positive prayer. The substance is not inert; it's responding to the thoughts and beliefs, the energy, being sent to it. I want the medicine to be filled with love and God-like wisdom, and I trust, believe, and know, that will happen through my efforts.

Later, after Mom has gone, when the last dose is being hung at 10 PM, I ask John if he wants to join me in my prayer ceremony. He earnestly accepts. We sit together on my hospital bed, the lights dim and gentle music playing. We both hold the double plastic bag in our hands, our heads bowed in reverence. I speak aloud, infusing the chemo with the intention of my prayer. Each time I affirm an intention of the medicine, John says in a whisper, "Yes." As I finish I look up at him, our faces just a foot from one another. We smile knowingly and I say, "And so it is."

He says, "Right on." I'm strengthened by his humbleness.

The treatment is going remarkably well. I have a PET scan half way through the six chemo treatments. The oncologist bounces into the exam room. She reports, "There's no cancer left anywhere! I had hoped for 80% improvement, which would have been terrific. This is miraculous!" While this sort of recovery can occur in patients who don't have a compromised immune system, the fact that my immune system has been depleted for decades makes this news more unusual. I'm already cancer-free!

But as I must complete the full chemotherapy regimen, I of course continue my meditations, prayers, work–outs at the gym and at home, and eating a fresh, healthy diet. Brent and I do fist pumps and high fives, smiling with jubilant embraces each time I complete a treatment. But it's complicated and what's perfect one day can turn to disaster the next. My medical teams and I have to balance chemo, keep my organs working, eliminate the cancer, and at the same time prevent potentially lethal infection. What's good for one condition is wrong for another.

I meet with my transplant surgeon. He's solemn but optimistic. He is already looking ahead to when the chemotherapy is done. He explains, "We have to get you back on a full immune suppression regimen right away. We lose transplanted organs because people wait too long after the final chemo is given before starting a full immune suppression dose. You need to see me within one or two weeks of your last chemo run to make sure your transplants are well-protected."

My survival was a tiny hole in a thin needle that I had to pass through, but at least there was an opening. I was two-thirds through the eye of the needle when the whole thing started to crumble.

Lying on the bed in our guest room in mid-July, I'm limp with exhaustion. I've slept most of the afternoon, but my limbs still feel too heavy for me to lift. Brent takes my temperature: 102 F—way too high and a sure sign of an infection somewhere. A CT of my chest is done. The oncologist sees multiple lesions throughout my lungs. "You have pneumonia," she tells me, "but we need to figure out what kind." My body stiffens with knowing concern. Pneumonia can kill a transplant patient, and now I'm a transplant patient who's also a cancer patient in the middle of receiving chemotherapy, which destroys one's infection-fighting cells. If it doesn't kill, it may lead to the need to be on a respirator. I also know that certain kinds of pneumonia are more lethal than others. Bacterial pneumonia can be treated with antibiotics. Viral pneumonia is a different problem and harder to treat, and the worst-case, pneumocystis pneumonia, often takes people to their graves.

I was admitted to the university hospital. After the tests, four doctors from the pulmonary and oncology departments stood beside my bed. "You have pneumocystis pneumonia." I feel my heart shake. It's the worst possible scenario. My lungs are full of thousands of nodules. They are taking up my air space. My oxygen saturation levels fall from a normal 100% to 80%, a severe impairment. My critical care nurse knowledge kicks in. *If I get too bad, I will need to be put on a respirator. If I can't recover my lungs, I could be on it for the rest of my life,* I think with dread. I have seen patients transferred to a permanent respirator facility. Often these patients are young, younger than me, and they have a life in an institution to look forward to. To me, this is not life; it's prison. It's torture. This would be an oppression too great for me. I'd rather die. I already have too many restrictions, too many limitations in my life that I'm managing on an hourly basis.

I center into my core, the place in me that remains solid and hopeful. I envision the outcome I want and keep all of my thoughts focused in that direction.

I'm started on massive doses of multiple types of antibiotics. Days go by. My fevers spike, then fall. I'm put on oxygen. As a nurse, I do self-prescribed lung exercises, forcing air into my lungs as much as possible. I start on another medicine that makes me terribly ill. The days are exceedingly long with little change in my status. I'm tired and sick. I'd rather just relax, but I watch the clock to do the breathing exercises and push myself through the fevers and vomiting at the same time. I force myself to stand up and walk the few paces of my hospital room, exercising my lungs, pushing myself to breathe deeply. I meditate and pray, staying focused on my successful recovery. It is hard work. In time, my fevers stabilize and my oxygen levels stay above 90% without supplemental oxygen. I'm released from the hospital but need to continue on the medication to continue treating the pneumonia. I'm warned, "This drug can cause kidney failure; we have to watch you closely." Seriously, I can't help but roll my eyes. I lift my upturned hand and tip my head. "Whatever," I say. Brent and I walk hand-in-hand from the hospital knowing full well this story is far from over.

After only a few more days, the now twice-weekly lab tests showed that my kidney is failing. I had to stop the medicine to go on a different one and hope that it worked as well to treat the aggressive pneumonia.

Since the chemo was on hold because of the pneumonia, I wasn't getting the immune suppression I needed for my organ transplants. Since my transplant surgeon had warned me about waiting too long to start my immune suppressants, I called the transplant clinic and alerted them. I pressed them to start my medication. The transplant team resisted saying my labs were stable. They didn't consult with my usual doctor. I'm unimpressed with their plan. I have a sense I ought to be doing something different.

Within the span of three days my pancreas function changed from normal to terrible. I was furious! I was in full-blown pancreas rejection, again. I had worked doggedly to maintain my pancreas after the first rejection. I was fighting like hell to build dams to keep the waters back and survive cancer and pneumonia. I wanted someone to be held accountable. But what does that matter? I feel bombarded, betrayed, and too small to conquer all of this.

My body is not youthful. I had had diabetes for decades. I have heart disease and I've lived on borrowed organs for almost thirty years. I know I'm resilient, but all of this makes me tired just thinking about the work it takes: mind, body, and spirit. And yet, I can't let my real fatigue overwhelm my determination.

Just as when I had kidney cancer four years ago, when I had the first pancreas rejection, I can't take the usual treatment course to try to reverse the rejection. The chemotherapy is on hold so I can try to recover from pneumonia. Somehow, my body is supposed to endure this and still survive. My spirit is not dissuaded. If there is even a fading shadow of a chance to come through this, I am determined to find that slim chance and breathe more life into it!

The rejection treatment is harsh. I'm already taking large doses of steroids to treat lymphoma, but they are now increased exponentially. The steroids give me what I call, 'Roid-rage." They make me feel like I'm being controlled by an outside force. My exhaustion is instantly replaced with anxiety and jitters. I feel what I'd imagine a heroin addict feels when a fix is needed. Sleeping is a monumental struggle each night. I am intolerant and can't stand myself. I don't know how Brent can put up with me. I become demanding and inconsolable, my emotions fluctuating from minute to minute. My thoughts are jumbled. I'm sleep deprived. I'm ravenous with a hunger that cannot be filled. I'm swollen from my eyelids to my toes, which makes me distraught and even more annoyed. As I endure all this in addition to the pneumonia and cancer, I get more and more angry. I feel myself boiling inside, thinking hateful, blaming, and judgmental thoughts. One night I erupt– screaming at Brent, then falling into sobs. I'm only a person. I'm not an ascended being. I honestly do need help. But what sort of help? No one can fight through the day for me. No one can become my body, taking on the experience for me.

One day Beth says to me, "I think it's time for you to cash in on some of that love you spread to so many, Shelli." Beth is right. She recalls the back patio healing circle she attended five years ago when my pancreas first met trouble. She organizes another such circle.

It's a beautiful July evening. A perfect, gentle breeze blows the soothing tepid air. In the bright blue sky, white, wispy clouds drift carefree. I've heard from many of my friends from across the world who say they will be with me in spirit tonight to pray for my total recovery.

Inside me, my insecure, little girl voice who believed her needs were less important mingles with my adult voice. *People are busy; it's a week night. Realistically many people just can't come. What if they think I'm a bother? I should really just do this on my own – no one else is really all that interested.* The thoughts weave in and out of my mind. I do my best to push the small voices down and remember the healed parts of myself.

Tonight people begin to drift down the sidewalk, through the tall trees to our back patio. I'm sitting crossed legged on my treatment table we've moved beneath the big oak tree. To my amazement, a long receiving line begins to form. I'm flabbergasted to find our patio packed with over seventy-five people who have come to pray and lift me up with their presence and hands.

There is something visceral, magical, about the presence of another, especially at a time of difficulty. More than reading a note on a card (which is terrific) or seeing a posting on social media offering love, the personal connection of someone's hands on mine, my heart touching theirs in an embrace, is remarkably affirming. The power of being witnessed validates my experience. I feel loved. The sense of being loved solidifies my commitment to live and gives me the resolve to carry on. I feel myself as a member of a community responsible for one another. I'm not doing this alone! The power of presence is immeasurable. Its transformative capacity is irreplaceable.

That night we had a beautiful ritual of healing that included all faiths, beliefs and ways of thinking. The essential element was that we were united together, all aligning with the truth that we are all a part of a single "Source." My friends and family symbolically lifted large rocks that had been placed around me on my treatment table. As they lifted them away, passing them to the next person, I heard, "You don't have to carry this burden alone; we are here to help you." People brought poems, uplifting messages and mostly, their authentic open hearts and honest love for me. The experience was renewing and shifted something within me! An everyday miracle occurred that night, in ways that went beyond improving my physical and emotional stamina. Those who attended also experienced a healing and they told me as much. "I'm not sure what just happened here, but you gave me such a healing," one friend remarked. I knew what it was. It was the sense of being a part of a community with no objective other than to be united in giving love, and in the giving came an unanticipated receiving. After just two days I was able to go for walks and again participate in household tasks.

In short order, my pancreas was once again miraculously salvaged. The pneumosystis pneumonia ebbed, though it took a year to resolve and I will need preventative medication for the rest of my life, which will be a very long time! I continued with the rest of the chemo treatments, physically stretched but emotionally bolstered by the healing circle that July evening.

I need another PET scan four weeks after I finish the last chemo treatment. Even though I had a scan that was clear of cancer already, the cancer can return, even during the treatment.

It's a warm evening in early September. I finished chemo three weeks ago. I'm in my bathroom when my fingers land on a single, enlarged node on my torso. I gasp. Horror runs through me and my legs weaken. The response is automatic. *Will this ever end?* Part of me is freaking out and another part is remembering all I've learned about my connection with God. Since I'm not ascended, the part of me that is scared and angry calls Beth. I rage and cry furiously with her over the phone.

Five minutes later, I'm laughing. She's laughing. In this moment, I need to honestly admit to and express my doubtful, tired, human side. After my tantrum, I have more capacity for the essence of my soul to dominate my thoughts. That night I step into my soul of love, and lean on my faith.

Finding the nodule prompted me to call to schedule my post-chemo PET scan. I schedule my post-chemo PET scan and oncologist visit for later that week.

At the oncology clinic Dr. Holtan opens the door and before she has fully entered the room she says, "Your PET scan is totally normal!" I look at her in silence. I smile. What I feel is relief, not because there's no cancer in my body, but because I'm affirmed in my belief. A single tear glides down my cheek. I turn and look at Brent. I wish so desperately I was able to see his face at this moment. I feel temporary grief that splinters ecstasy.

He says in his unshakable confidence, "I told you."

I jump up and ardently first hug Brent, then Dr. Holtan. She returns my embrace with no inhibition. "You told me a cure was possible!"

She replies, "You had me going several times. This type of pneumonia kills healthy people. The organ rejection on top of the chemo is seldom a good outcome. You had a very aggressive type of lymphoma." I sit with myself, taking in the enormity of what I had gone through for the last several months. As each potentially fateful event occurred, while individually challenging, I had been able to manage to isolate each so the enormity didn't cripple me. And when it did feel too much, I asked for help. Now, listening to Dr. Holtan compress the experience into a few minutes, I felt immeasurable gratitude: for my faith, my blessings and for my tenacity.

"You're the strongest person I know," Dr. Holtan says to me. I shy away from her compliment. "You see a lot of people here, lots of really sick people," I say to her. "Yes, I do," she says, her resolute gaze not moving from my face. "And I'm telling you, you are the strongest person I know."

I'm the strongest person I know, too.

THE HEALING

When I was diagnosed with lymphoma, I knew I was being given a choice: Choose life or death. It was as though the universe was saying,

"Is your physical life still worth living?" I did seriously consider whether or not I still had the will to endure. To keep the desire to live burning, I need a reason to keep going, to maintain my earthly existence despite future physical trials. I looked back at the medical situations of my life that felt absurd to me, and I wondered if I wasn't tired of it all, or if I wanted to carry on. I realized I had to own my yet unrealized reason for living, and move forward with unwavering commitment. Without a reason to live, I felt that surviving cancer, and whatever else would come my way, was hopeless.

When I am hopeless I lose my connection to a meaningful existence. I lose the connection to my soul. Without soul-attachment, I am left with only the limiting beliefs of my fears: fear of a hostile world that is joyless and unsafe, fear of being inadequate, and therefore, incapable of independence, fear of being controlled by events or others and therefore losing my identity, fear of being betrayed and therefore consumed with suspicion and mistrust, and fear of being imperfect and therefore, undeserving of love.

As I treated the lymphoma, I realized more healing of these fears was still possible and on a much different level than I had previously understood. I needed to let my soul lead my life, not my fears or my ego. The only way I could live as my Soul was to accept my human fears, not deny them or try to destroy them. I had to embrace them and all of the past events that led me to feel these fears. Paradoxically, the more I embraced my fear, the more it lost its power and began to shrink. As fear dissolved, love emerged. In the presence of love, I felt completely peaceful, confident, and faithful. I knew that I was, and would always be, okay.

The more I accepted that this could be my final chapter, how my life story ended, the more my fear that the cancer would kill me began to leave my daily thoughts. I actually grew stronger with more resolve. My faith deepened and I soon began to feel invincible.

The strength didn't come from me. It came from the open space that was created when I let go of resisting my fear. When I resisted fear, the energy in my body closed, shut down, and there was no place for my Soul and God to reside. Accepting my fears relaxed my mind and body, which made a space for Love to enter and spread. As the Love spread, there was less space for malignancy: malignant thoughts and malignant cells.

I believe prayer travels on the energy of Love. I believe the answer to the many prayers said on my behalf was that I accepted myself as unconditional Love and innately worthy of receiving favor. In Love, my faith is resolute and through my faith I can receive the healing energy of prayer. My spiritual growth had taught me that so long as I saw myself as damaged, unworthy, deserving of punishment, and laden with guilt, Love's blessing would not, could not, enter. There could be no healing, no miracle. Faith and hope and love abide, the Bible says, but the greatest of these is love. How simple can it get?

Cancer was my quintessential opportunity to live as Source: to think, breathe, *be,* my Soul. Ultimately, it was about completely redefining how I saw myself in relationship to God. I needed to accept the truth that God and I are not separate, but unified. And in that unification I realized that since God is unconditional Love, then so must there also be that potential in me.

The idea of changing how I self-identified was daunting, even in the presence of a lethal illness. A part of me wanted to maintain my beliefs about myself, people, and how I was told the world worked. I wanted to be able to think of myself as "only human" so I wouldn't have the responsibility that came with living as my Soul. I was intimidated. *What if I can't do it?* I asked myself. *Have I then failed? Will this be an ultimate life lesson that I end up botching? How would I know that I'd arrived when I wasn't exactly sure where I was going? How would I know if I'd accomplished my task? And what if, in the process of living as my*

Soul, I end up losing key components that define me as a singularly unique individual?

When I heard myself asking these questions I had a very real experience of my personality talking to my Soul. My personality is the part of me that felt incapable and unsure and is associated with my ego. The small me was talking and the bigger me responding. My personality was having a conversation with The Divine. It was vividly real and created a quantum shift in me. That shift was a single step across a thin, white line. It was very minute and simplistic, but powerful.

I was transformed in another way as I learned the lessons that came bundled in the package of cancer. I came to understand that all healing is about transformation, transcendence, and finally, transfiguration.

In transformation, I change the meaning of the traumatic events in my life from just sorrow to include lessons and greater wisdoms. In transcendence, I rise above my previous judgments, coping strategies, and limited view of how life works. And in transfiguration, a process I'm only just beginning, I change from being identified only as a body with flesh, blood and an ego that wants to reign supreme, to a kinesthetic experience of being also Spirit, Soul, and Source. This is more than an intellectual understanding. Transfiguration is a kinesthetic, tangible experience of being everything all at once, flesh, organs, personality, and being Infinite.

Through cancer, I transcended from a faith system that was based on thoughts and ideas, to a tangible inner experience of my Divinity. This inner experience of myself as Divine allows me to feel joy despite life's difficulties. I have to be willing to recognize the existence of joy; it doesn't come and announce itself in the quagmire of traumatic events. I've always known that I am the author of my life by the way I respond to all events, both trials and triumphs. Yet in living as my Soul, I feel an even more profound ability to access joy, passion, and love. I imagine it's like having a cataract removed; joy, passion, and love have always been present and I could feel them, experience them, but as my Soul everything became more intense and vivid.

Through lymphoma I realized that I could not master my fear with my will or positive affirmations. I couldn't extinguish its voice only by analyzing it. I couldn't move beyond the righteousness of my ego's demands by pretending to be loving and compassionate, all the while merely gagging the voice inside me that wanted to scream out criticism and hostility. Each individual past awareness was absolutely necessary for me to take my next step in spiritual development. I couldn't start with living as my soul. I found no irony in the fact that my life had been a series of difficult medical and emotional trials that became more complex until I was struck with a systemic cancer.

I know that the illnesses are linked to my spiritual development, or at least that's the way I view them now. I didn't see them that way when they were first happening. Certainly by the time of my double organ transplant, I saw that there was a connection. Now I tie my illnesses and life traumas to spiritual maturation and healing, at least that's what I decided to do with them. I don't see my challenges or illnesses as direct insults from God, but rather, a course I could use to bring me closer to God . I suppose I could have viewed my illnesses as only struggles. I could have seen my stories as unfair or only tragic, but this thought process leaves me a victim. I truly believe the gift is within the tragedy, but I must find it. The culmination of all of my past healings and learnings led me to a place where I was spiritually conscious enough to live as Soul-embodied.

In order to live as my Soul I first needed to understand what my Soul is. Likely you've read the word "soul" throughout this book and passed by it believing you understand the word. But do you understand the truth of what your Soul really is or why you have one? Could you discuss its nature with others? Is your understanding of the Soul based on descriptors that are open for interpretation yet you see as absolutes?

Have you spent time in quiet contemplation feeling, being acquainted with your Soul?

I spent many years, decades really, contemplating the nature of the soul. I studied and researched with theologians, took college courses, studied spiritual scriptures, and prayed and meditated. At various times throughout my searching, I felt contented and comfortable with my conclusions. Then, another life experience would occur, or I'd gain more wisdom through my contemplative mind, and what I had understood about the Soul morphed into something different. The change was always additive. In other words, the nature of my understanding of the Soul grew upon my previous understandings. Eventually, I became adept at being able to discern my personality from my Soul.

If you delve into your own inner experience of learning who you are as your Soul rather than your personality, you will eventually discover what I did: that the Soul feels and talks and moves and lives much differently than does our personality. I invite you to open your contemplative mind. Find stillness so that you know your Soul. The one thing I will suggest as being universally true is that the Soul, if left to its own accord and not distorted by our ego personality, is unconditional Love.

Most of us don't recognize unconditional Love because it is so rare to experience this amount of purity. People are imperfect. Most of us can say we love someone unconditionally. The love we have for our children is often defined in this way. But when we become angered with our children or loved ones, it's fairly common to close our heart center, even for a moment. Humans are generally perceptive. Even if we don't interpret the change in our brain, we automatically sense the change energetically. And so the idea of truly experiencing unconditional Love is not commonplace.

The real experiences of being both inside and outside of my physical body gave me a tangible vantage point from which to form my understandings about the nature of the soul. Finally, when I was diagnosed with a potentially fatal cancer, I was able to meld together all of my past experiences with my past study and contemplation. What I arrived at is an awareness that the soul is the single, unique droplet of the Divine, of God, of the ultimate Creator, that is individually Me. Just as a single droplet of water is still the ocean, but is not the entire ocean, so is my soul still the essence of God, but is not all of God. The droplet of ocean water has all the same salts and minerals and properties of the ocean; it doesn't look or feel like lake water or pond water; it remains ocean water. So, my Soul, as I see it, is the Me that is exactly the same composition as God. And Source is the body from which my Soul, all Souls, are born. And since Source is only Love, then, too, my Soul is also only Love in its purest form. Our personalities can interfere with our Souls' desire, its intention to live as Love. But this distortion only appears in the physical realm where personality and ego reside. In the spirit realm, we have no ego, no personality, and all Souls are nothing other than the purity of Love that Source created them to be.

People talk about "soul" and "spirit." Often times I find the words are used interchangeably. But I think they are very different. Soul seems to be the permanent part of one's identity. I think of it as the template of who we are as individuals. Soul has the identity of being Love. The Soul has a plan.

Spirit on the other hand, I see as the energy, or the fuel, that allows the Soul to live out its plan. The Spirit doesn't have a plan of manifestation on its own. Instead, our Spirit is the very breath that allows our Soul to manifest as Love on earth. Returning to the Hebrew word (which is spelled in various ways in English), Rukha. This word means both spirit and breath. So consider then, any time you use the word "spirit" you might substitute the word "breath." Breath is the first essential element of life. Without breath, without spirit, life cannot happen. Soul cannot happen. When we take our first *inspiration,* we bring our Soul into the physical. When we take our last *expiration,* our Soul exits the physical and returns home.

Living as my Soul, I began to live more fully as Love. My purpose became to serve Love's purpose. In other words, to serve God's purpose.

The only way I could master fear was to be Love, to hold Love in the cells of my body, every cell, even malignant cells, and let the amazing restorative power of Love impart its divine healing. Without my full acceptance of self as Love, I remain a prisoner to all of my self-doubts as well as my self-righteousness. I believe my misconceptions. I languish in the belief that I'm ill. When I recognize that I am Love itself, I'm able to experience a transpersonal relationship between me and The Creator, Source, God – whatever name defines that which is indefinable. When I experience myself as Love, disease, strife, and judgments all vanish from my reality. What remains is irrevocable faith, stillness, and eternal peace. In this state I'm able to just be without thinking or doing.

Buddha said, "To live is to suffer," and, "Find joy in all things." This is the paradox of life and the crux of the healing process. We are charged to somehow endure the audacity of life and also be able to marry this reality with our soul that uses each moment for our evolution.

Our goal in healing is to live as a Soul on earth, not to aspire to ascension. In fact, if we believe we have ascended, we likely need to reconsider. Ascension disregards and disrespects the human experience. Most of the time ascension is an attempt to escape the body and live in an unsustainable spiritual fantasy. The idea of ascension implies that we believe our spiritual self is superior to our physical self.

Living as our Soul is different than ascension. Instead of moving out of the body, we move more fully into the body as our living Souls. Here we understand that divinity is not outside the physical body, but rather, embedded within the Soul which is centered deeply in the heart. It is not centered in the brain. It doesn't have its origin in our thoughts and beliefs. This is the home of our ego. When we live Soul-embodied, we have more, not less, contact with our physical nature. We feel the body more fully. We experience our emotions more fully. We have greater intuition and general awareness of our surroundings. When our bodies and minds are imbued with the energy of our Souls, we are saturated with endless Love and this becomes how we experience life, which is dramatically different than how we experience life from the perspective of our egos.

The process starts by beginning to become honest with ourselves. We admit and own all the ways that we are hurting, all the ways in which we fight and are cruel or callous. Next we change our old ways of coping, thinking, and behaving to healthier habits and beliefs. And finally we experience the self as both wholly physical and spiritual. This is how we become Soul-embodied and how we shift from an external experience of God to an internal, visceral experience.

We don't need to be dealing with physical catastrophes to experience life as unfulfilling or strenuous. Living as Soul and discovering limitless Love, can feel impossible when ordinary life is so damn difficult. This is one reason why ascension is generally not the goal for ordinary people. True healing, meaningful healing, lasting healing, always begins with validation of our present and past situations. We will never follow a mentor who denies the truth of our human experience. We want mentors who value and validate our suffering and difficulties. We want our mentors to be human just like us.

When we heal our stories and move into the contemplative mind, we begin to change our views about suffering and contentment. Our challenge, if we are seeking to live Soul-embodied, is to be able to accept the injustice of life and still see the beauty of the moment and be encouraged about the future. This optimistic viewpoint requires resiliency.

Resiliency is an interesting characteristic that has been well-studied. Some people seem to be innately endowed with the capacity to spring back time after time. For most people, though, resiliency is a character trait that's developed. The more we are faced with situations that ask us to rebound, the more our resiliency develops. In fact, over time, if we are the type of person who uses tragedy to our advantage, we can become nearly immune to future collapse each time we encounter disaster and survive. These types of people can actually use difficulties as a desirable occurrence.

Not everyone will develop a feeling of invincibility. Some people will feel dazed and shattered by even the most miniscule turbulence. It's even more important for these individuals to recognize that although their lives have been disrupted, hope for a better tomorrow is within reach and is possible through the healing process.

By the time lymphoma struck me I had learned that I was an "overcomer." Certainly, the multiple "near misses" I had encountered bolstered my resiliency. But more accurately, it was my faith that grew. I had deliberately utilized the medical and emotional challenges of my life as a tool for changing my emotional, mental, and physical health. I learned I had to rely on faith because everything else was transient. When I was faced with an illness that could kill me very quickly, I had arrived at a new pinnacle of healing. I became centered on my spiritual maturation, the health of my consciousness, my soul, and my union with the Creator to a depth I hadn't previously touched.

Despite our modern-day technologies and conveniences, ours is a culture that is more unsatisfied, unhappy, and unfulfilled than ever before. We feel little peace and there is no reprieve. We are bombarded with distractions that pull us away from our Souls. We've sold out reflective prayer to searching the internet for answers. We go to bed with worrisome thoughts about tomorrow; whether to pay the electric or the phone bill, trying to devise a way to be in three places at once, knowing that every breath will be a struggle, with our pain still shredding our ravaged hearts and minds. Although most of us living in industrialized nations are not burdened by having to chop wood to cook, tote water on our shoulders to drink, or hunt for our food, we are a civilization that reports increased stress, pressure, and unhappiness. These are the reasons why we need something greater than the fleeting and demanding moment surrounding us to sustain us.

We have pushed silence aside. We've forgotten the contemplative mind that people relied on for centuries. We have forgotten how to be quiet and alone with ourselves. Similarly, we have let go of meaningful community and the time when showing up in someone's moment of crisis or need was expected instead of being out of the ordinary. Our priorities have changed so that our individual needs most often take precedence over the needs of others, even if that person is helpless in that moment. It's not that we ought to negate our own needs; it's the heart-fullness with which we respond to others that makes the difference.

When it comes right down to it, most of us don't want to invest in the work it takes to consider our souls. We don't see the value or necessity of learning about our injured egos so that we can live as our authentic selves. We would rather play bridge or shop or watch baseball. And I understand why: life is already demanding and difficult. We want to have fun when we have free time, not develop our Soul-nature.

The truth is, we can do both.

We need to return to Love. Love is who we truly are. We have found little sustainability through anything other than a deeply penetrating experience of knowing who we are in our souls and feeling a personal connection with something larger than ourselves.

At this point we are entering a level of healing that goes beyond particular events, emotions or thoughts. Earlier we needed to find purpose in order to access our joy, our passion, and our connection to the grand scheme of things. When we reach the stage of soul-embodiment and spiritual maturation, our specific purpose becomes less important. What we seek now is the ability to simply *be* in the world. Instead of "What will I do?" we begin to ask, "How shall I be?" When we purposely seek how to be, we are moving into a state of greater enlightenment, a state beyond transforming our thinking, beliefs, and pain. We are entering the transfiguration process. This process continues for the rest of our lifetimes.

We are challenged, for those who want this level of healing, to live and think as the Soul, which has, as its only identification, boundless love. In this stage of healing we desire a life experience that is less attached to outcomes and is more concerned with being able to see all events as opportunities for our Souls to grow.

We need to focus on nourishing our Souls rather than our gluttonous egos, which are never satiated anyway. One way to begin to operate from our Souls is to ask, *What would Love do?* We need to discern whether our loving acts originate in our Souls or our egos.

Many people do loving things, which is good, but not all good actions emanate from the Soul. Some acts of love come from ego. Loving acts that come from the ego always have an underlying intention to maintain our image, to gain favor with our peers and employers, society in general, or a doctrinal guideline. Loving acts that originate from the ego are always attached to a desired outcome. These sorts of loving actions set us up to feel angry if the outcome we hoped for doesn't come to fruition. "I gave all this time and money and you didn't change a thing!" Our egos feel betrayed and disrespected. Ego-based love expects reciprocity. "If I do good for you, you will do good for me."

Acts of love that rise from the Soul have no attachment to outcome. Soul-based love is unfamiliar because we have been conditioned to believe we are our egos and not our Souls. We find it difficult to give love with no expectation or need for reciprocity, because this is what the ego is accustomed to. When our actions are based in love but we have no attachment or expectation, we know we are acting from our Souls.

Each of your stories provides wisdom for you to enhance your Soul expression and tame your ego's insistence on being the driver of your life. Your greatest peace and freedom is grounded in your *be-ing*. Let go of focusing on what you do and instead, focus on your *intention* for doing what you do. Pause and ask yourself, "Do I wish to be my ego or my Soul in this moment?" What's important is not which you choose, but that you are aware of your choice.

It is possible to live in the world focused on our Souls and still be responsible people. Soul-embodied people aren't eternally meditating in a world of euphoria; they still operate within the law, earn honest money, and contribute more than they take. They've simply realized that the ego is not their true identity.

We can teach in a loving way. We can express opinions and beliefs in a loving way. We can achieve justice in a loving way. Rise every morning and know that you are nothing other than love; every cell, every thought is love. Anything that doesn't feel like love needs to be healed. When we begin to scatter all that is not love to the wind, we organically experience the truth of who we have always been. Instead of seeing your story as breaking you, realize it has been purposely orchestrated to break you open.

You are what you have been seeking.

"Someday, after mastering winds, waves, tides, and gravity, we shall harness the energy of love; and for the second time in the history of the world, man will have discovered fire."

Pierre Teilhard de Chardin

"True love is inexhaustible; the more you give, the more you have. And if you go to draw at the true fountainhead, the more water you draw, the more abundant is its flow."

Antoine de Saint-Exupery

"The Soul is intended but for one thing: to love and be loved."

Shelli Stanger Nelson

"Love cannot be said."

Rumi

"Every act in the universe comes from love. Those that do not are a crying out for help."

Gregory David Roberts

"How long will you worry about making a living? How long will you pamper your body, stuff your mouth, throat and belly? How long should you bust your jaws and teeth? Worry about your soul for a moment."

Rumi

Chapter Nine

THE PROCESS OF BECOMING

ONCE I WAS DIVORCED I SAW AN OPEN SPACE FOR ME. IT WAS MY chance to discover the real me. I was unsure of who I was, what I valued or desired in life, how I should behave, and even how to react in social situations. Even in my late 30's, I questioned the right way to greet someone. I was uncertain if I should gush when I heard of a terrible tragedy, or offer quiet sympathy. I questioned what style of clothes I liked and if it was "okay" for me to wear particular fashions. I wasn't sure if I was a tough rock and roller or a tender pacifist. I often found myself agreeing with opposing viewpoints depending on who I was with at the time. I didn't trust my opinions because I seldom had my opinions validated.

I was bursting to break free from the pre-set definitions I felt were imposed on me by being someone's daughter, someone's wife and someone who was blind. I wanted to run away from the expectations I felt living in an upper middle class, predominately white suburb of the homogeneous Midwest. Now divorced from my first husband, as a grown, single woman, I was exhilarated with the thought that I didn't have to explain myself to anyone.

In August of 1994, now six months into my separation from Tom, I begin my first sweep at defining myself. I leave my suburban home and my average job as a nurse in a hospital, my average day-to-day experiences, and set out across the country in the front seat of a Cadillac. I'm with Bobby, the married man with whom I'm having an affair, and his seventy-year-old uncle from New York. All three of us are squeezed into the front seat as we travel. I've never been to the infamous motorcycle rally in Sturgis before, and that's why I'm here.

I'm standing on the sidewalk in a black leather halter-top covered with fringe and beads, black boots and black leather shorts, which are cut more like panties. The leather has been totally cut from the rear of the shorts and replaced by thin, purple lace covering my butt cheeks. I'm drinking a bottle of beer. I've drunk probably less than a dozen in my thirty-two years, and I'm posing for a group of men taking my photo. I feel hot, seductive, dangerous, edgy, rebellious, and, *undefined*. I love it!

Once the door to freedom was opened, I took every opportunity to try on many roles and beliefs, wondering if I could find myself in any of them. I did things and tried things that were exceptionally out of character for me. The decision to have an affair with a married man went against my values. But at the time, I didn't realize what my values even were. The severe injustice I felt by being betrayed by my husband and close friends made me rebellious and reckless. If others could be self-absorbed, uncontrolled and immoral, then so could I!

I desperately needed to understand who I was as an individual separate from who I was in my family and in society. I longed to live as myself and not capitulate to what was all around me or who I was taught to be. It was a need so desperate that if I couldn't achieve it, there was no sense in my being alive, because I wasn't living *my* life. If I couldn't fully individuate, I knew my spirit would be crushed and I would live a meaningless life of pretense.

I didn't desire a "nice" life. I wanted a life that permitted me to be blatantly myself. I didn't feel the need to totally disassociate from my work, family and community. Rather, my quest was how to be myself *within* my traditional community and my family.

I struggled to find my inner authority and sense of justice-based power. I felt powerless in preventing the destruction of my body. I felt ineffectual in my marriage. I felt very small in my parents' home. Yet I also felt pressure to grow up fast. In doing so, I took on responsibilities that were beyond my capability. One of those tasks was managing diabetes. I felt pressured to make mature decisions even though I was a child, an adolescent and a young adult. In my attempt to find my inner authority and right-sized power, I floundered.

I often felt a need to be right. It seemed to me that there were two positions on any topic: right or wrong. Wrong not only meant I was inaccurate, but that I had failed. I felt my failure made me powerless and at risk of being relentlessly criticized. In an attempt to avoid criticism, I often felt a desperate need to defend myself and to hide my errors, what I felt were shortcomings and failures. My insecurity and lack of self-identity couldn't tolerate being seen this way. My strategy was to lie. I felt afraid of not knowing, of being wrong. Making things up gave me a temporary sense of safety. But when my safety came from my deception, I felt disempowered and a like fraud. I was stuck, with no way to win.

As a woman I felt less significant than my male counterparts. While men could be defined and admired for a variety of traits and talents, the messages I heard from society and at home were that my attractiveness and sensuality were the most important qualities I had as a woman. At times, being known as those qualities made me feel good about myself, but more often they made me feel inferior to men. I struggled with two opposing viewpoints: wanting to be accepted by and desirable to men, yet also wanting to be seen and valued as more than just a face and a body. As a normal female adolescent I was searching for a healthy self-definition that included my sexuality. And then, at sixteen, I was raped outside our suburban home.

I'm jogging in our neighborhood. It's after 10 P.M. I've waited until dark because I feel clumsy, too big with my curvy body. I'm not an athlete. I'm not a good runner. I lumber along on the sidewalks and streets. It's strenuous. I feel as though I'm running through mud. My blood sugar isn't stable, and that makes the vigorous exercise even more difficult. But I want to keep going. I believe I will be more acceptable with slimmer thighs and a smaller rear end. More boys will find me attractive and therefore, worthy of love and thus, confirming my value. I want to be athletic. I know Dad admires athletes. I want to please him more than anything.

The night is misty and a drizzly rain falls. The heavy summer heat has thankfully been replaced by less humid and cooler September air. The darkness feels solid around me. The streets are deserted. The houses are quiet; front porches and yard chairs are empty. As I jog past them, I feel alone and without allies. Some houses sit dark and lonely, with no sign of people. Others have the drapes pulled and I see cozy amber lights shining from behind them. I feel comforted when I see a lit home. On one hand, I feel safe that no one can see me. But my sense of protection is vastly overshadowed by my terror. My eyes dart all around, searching the dark corners of the houses, the sides of the buildings, and the depths of the bushes for skulking dangers.

I'm almost finished with the mile run. I'm within one short block of our house. As I run, I notice a man walking on my side of the street through the drizzling rain. He's walking hastily toward me; he's wearing jeans and a hooded jacket. The hood is tied tightly over his head. Both of his hands are thrust into his jacket pockets.

The distance between me and the stranger quickly closes. Suddenly, my mind says, *Turn! This isn't right!* By the time I finish my thought we are side-by-side.

"Stop right there," the dark stranger says in an authoritative voice. Stunned, I stop and stare immobile into the barrel of a gun pointed straight at me.

Confused thoughts flash unorganized through my mind. I'm standing only seven feet from him. He doesn't move. Neither do I. The sight of a gun being purposely aimed at my body is beyond my comprehension. I try reasoning with him.

"You can't do this," I say with a quavering voice. Pointing at my home I tell him, "I live right there." I force my eyes away from the nose of the pistol the stranger is holding with a double-fisted grip. To my left, across the street and one house away from me, is my home.

I look at the front of our house. The front door is open and the screen door is letting in the cool, night air. I watch my brother, Scott. He's sitting on the near end of the sofa. He's wearing his orange San Francisco T shirt. He's staring at the TV. I know he's watching a re-run of *The Rockford Files*. I watch him lift a potato chip and put it in his mouth.

I can't believe this is actually happening, that I can see the glow of the TV on my brother's face while a man is assaulting me at gunpoint. I'm frozen in sheer terror. I'm so scared I can't move, scream, or think. I'm sixteen years old.

The rapist tells me to walk toward him. "Quick, quick," he says. I walk robotically three steps in his direction. I feel disembodied.

The rapist snatches me and abruptly turns me away from him. Pressing my back firmly to his body, he holds a knife against my throat with one hand and pushes the nose of the pistol into my ribs with the other. "Don't look at me," he orders, "And do everything I say." I'm willing to do anything so he doesn't cut my throat or shoot me.

I was violated in ways I hadn't considered possible that night. I had no experience with sex or the acts he forced me to perform. My identity as a woman was in tatters. Was I safe to be a woman? Was I responsible for what happened because I'm a woman? Were my shorts and tank top inappropriate and seductive? From that moment forward the idea of me engaged in intimate encounters was dirty, disgusting, and shameful. More than that, *I* was dirty, disgusting and shameful. It took me many years, even into my second marriage, to fully process the event, and to separate who I AM from what I felt I was during the attack.

Defining myself as a woman in the context of my sexuality was one of the more difficult tasks of my becoming me. I was split between two conflicting beliefs: My sexuality is forbidden and filthy, and my value as a woman comes solely from being sexually desirable. I learned the place of the middle ground, so that today I own my feminine sexuality in a way that is a beautiful part of me instead of repulsive and shameful.

Before I began to develop more of my healthy, adult self, my injured self led my life. I erroneously thought, *This is who I am and my reactions are justified.* I was steeped in the pain of my child's story. I defended against having my legitimate needs not taken seriously, again. I defended against being mocked and teased, again. I defended against being controlled and feeling humiliated, again. I protected myself from feeling betrayed and my fear of being seen as insufficient, imperfect, and therefore, unworthy of gentleness and love, again.

I had pretended to be a warrior, afraid of nothing with no challenge too big. But the truth was I had an extremely tender and sensitive heart that I protected with my warrior. I pretended to be independent, that I didn't have needs, and I could do it all myself. But inside I felt deficient and afraid that if I had a need, it automatically implied I was needy. I sacrificed my own needs in favor of the more important needs of others.

I pretended to be confident, but inside I was insecure and felt most people would find me unsatisfactory. I believed people didn't like the real me, so I created a false front based on what I thought others wanted me to be. I unconsciously walked through a room saying, *Hi, I'm Shelli. Who do you need me to be?* This led to social anxiety and exhaustion.

As I healed, I became conscious of what I had been doing and what my fears were. I was able to figure out who I truly was, aside from who and what I felt I *ought* to be. I found my legitimate needs, my trust, and my unique abilities and talents. I allowed my innate ability to relate compassionately with others to be seen. I openly revealed my wisdom of teaching and leadership instead of staying small and covering my brilliance, so that others wouldn't feel threatened. What I found was my authentic self that burned inside. Instead of forcing myself to play small, stay low, keep quiet, I was able to find the courage I needed to be me regardless of the consequences. Ultimately, I learned to live as my Soul, not my thoughts and limiting beliefs about myself. I learned to disregard the roles and titles that had been put upon my back by others, and to choose my own title instead.

It was only after I accepted and expressed the truths of who I am at my core that I was able to authentically and lovingly embrace my community and my nuclear family. Instead of feeling forced to conform, now I can accept the uniqueness of others and myself. Instead of imposing my voice to be heard, I can listen to the voices of others while still hearing my own. Instead of needing to be right, I'm comfortable in my not knowing. And when I surrender, a myriad of possibilities appear. Instead of living in fear of being me, I am confident in who I am.

THE HEALING

The process of my becoming me took me a long time. I'm still honing my ability to be comfortable as myself and to show up without voices of self-doubt and insecurity echoing in my brain. Sometimes someone or something distresses me profoundly. When this happens, I forget I'm safe being me, and I can fall back into my habitual coping strategies from my early childhood. I believe that's just the way it works.

For the most part I have become a conscious adult who can live from a mature, higher-self place, one who has self-assurance and isn't afraid of authentic expression. If I have a bad day or am over stressed or weak from fatigue or worry, I might fall back to old patterns. The automatic negative thoughts kick in and suddenly I'm no longer with my friend or colleague; they've managed to morph into my critical parent or the most beautiful girl at my high school. My key learning has been to witness my emotional responses and behaviors and to make a purposeful decision to change them or not.

Becoming my authentic self has taught me to love my unique characteristics and to risk being me despite the possibility of disappointing others. I learned that living as myself, without hiding or suppressing or trying to be more or less than who I truly am, was the single most important healing achievement of my life. It wasn't the final healing, nor the most valuable, but the most essential, because without authenticity I was doomed to live a life based on the expectations and needs of others. If I didn't discover and live as me, the other healings were a sham: finding forgiveness, learning how to trust, reaching to live as my Soul.

Breaking away from the crowd or the norm of my family system meant I would likely face judgments and criticism from those people. This was hard at first. I still wanted their love and approval. Renouncing my truth, my soul, however, was too high a price to pay for others' acceptance. As I allowed myself to discover and be my authentic self, my integrity and my desire to be true to myself were much more gratifying and sustaining than the ceaseless craving for external validation. With time, the people who mattered, really mattered, came to accept me.

When I changed, the terms of many of my relationships changed as well. Most of my relationships strengthened, became more honest and fulfilling. Others dissolved. After the mourning process of losing some people who had been important in the past, I realized that those relationships had reached their sunset.

Today my relationships are more meaningful because I'm present, as myself, instead of acting, trying to think of the right answer, or wear the right clothes, or come up with the appropriate response. It takes courage for me to be who I truly am, to tell the truth of my story whole-heartedly, but each day that I show up as *me*, it gets easier.

The most critical thing I learned was to tolerate others' negative emotions and reactions. Sometimes my affable, open nature provokes others who believe I ought to be more subtle, less outspoken. Sometimes my tendency to be truthful makes people squirm, because I dare to say I was hurt or angry. I laugh and love with abandon. Sometimes my intensity offends those who believe that emotion is bad or scary (especially in the Scandinavian land of Minnesota, home of the "nice" people). I can still be tempted to please others and be who they want me to be, to make them more comfortable. But when I do, I betray myself, I dim my light, and then I feel repressed and resentful.

As I became more myself, I sometimes felt melancholy for what I'd left behind: a false identity I'd believed was me. A bit of me sometimes felt afraid, believing that my real identity meant I had to behave in a particular way all the time. I felt if I lived as my Soul, my true self, I had to surrender my irreverent humor, my wild side that loves to dance seductively, that curses, or gets angry. What I came to learn, though, is that these characteristics are just as sacred and holy as my sincerity and reverence for The Divine. In fact, my confidence in my connection with Divinity is what allows me to be both fully human with the full scope of human emotions and frailties along with my spiritual Divinity.

As I live my life as me, I find I have fewer judgments, fewer biases, less stress and discord. I experience more peace in me and around me.

It is hard to feel satisfied until we accept who we are at the depths of our being. I ached to experience myself as magnificent. I came to understand that we, all of us, are magnificent souls of light, products of a creation so inspired it took the mind of God to create us. As I emerged from my confusion, I realized the truth: there is nothing that can harm me, nothing that can dim my light, nothing that can leave me in millions of pieces so long as I can keep just one finger connected to the truth of who I am. I am the I Am before I was wounded.

I am no different than you. I'm not nearer to God, nor further away. I'm an average person who grew up average and later discovered her extraordinary living soul. We all start in the same place. We all start in a desert, or at the bottom of the sea, broken, with pieces of us missing. We can recover each missing part through the healing process. We can't move with grace; we can't experience delight; we can't live as our Souls until we have all of our parts recovered, repaired, and reclaimed as wholly ours.

What parts of yourself have been left behind, scattered about in your story? Some pieces may be chips. Others may be entire sections of your heart, or your spirit, your lucid mind, or your physical body. The idea of collecting all that is missing can feel overwhelming. The only thing you need to do today is to take one single step.Remember that healing our stories is not an instantaneous event. Our egos tend to want immediate fixes to magically restore us. Long-lasting changes don't usually happen this way. Sudden miracles sometimes occur that can only be explained as the hand of God. And sometimes the miracle takes ten months or ten years to arrive. Waiting ten years doesn't feel as glorious as an instantaneous miracle, but the soul doesn't care about that. Every step forward is miraculous in its own way.

It's typical to float just above the surface of the well that holds the fire of our trauma and misery, or mere discontent. Generally we dip a toe in, even wade in the heat and want to believe we have scorched all there is to be incinerated. We have to give ourselves time to burn all the wood that holds our fury and grief, confusion and loss, even if the woodpile keeps re-appearing year after year. If we don't, we get half a healing, and who wants that? Not me; I want my whole life. I want to feel my entire Soul! We need to pour out the entirety of our insanity-making thoughts, our twisted beliefs and emotions festering within our hearts and minds, so when we sew them back together we're starting with lush, fertile soil.

People tend to think that releasing emotions is injurious. Releasing our real emotions can be detrimental if we are attached to them, continually recycling them, causing us to collapse and not be able to function in life. We have a tendency to believe the pain is happening in this moment. It's not; the pain is what already happened. The emotional expression of this moment is the healing.

Burning all the wood, pouring out all that is suffering within you, begins a pilgrimage that leads to unbound forgiveness of whatever and whoever has tried to spoil your peace. Your work leads to a liberation and freedom to live in the present moment instead of being bound to your unhealed stories.

Pour out everything so that bitterness and hatred don't shrivel your spirit. Hold on to nothing. When you believe you are finished, start over again. Let your whole body express your anguish, with a trusted friend, a healer, a therapist, a tree, or the unseen companions at your side. Howl at the moon and shout to the seemingly empty heavens if that's what you need. Weep silent tears and rock your hurting heart. Admit to your terror of the process, and know your fear is only your unhealed self, trying to convince you not to take the risk.

Admit your stubbornness, your pride, and your worry of being inappropriate or wrong or looking like a fool. Own your judgments and biases, your indignation, and your shame. Recognize the voices that project onto you, their limitations and what it means to heal. Keep them far away.

Find a reason to believe, clench that single strand of hope, and do not let go. In time, it will become an entire tapestry.

Are you willing to take the risk? What do you have to lose? Better yet, what do you stand to gain?

My story is about unusual medical challenges that I saw as opportunities to heal physically, and in every aspect of health. I felt like the statue in the stone, and my would-be calamities were my motivation to persistently and deliberately chisel away all that wasn't me, so that I could have a happier, more meaningful way of living. Instead of ruining my spirit, I more fully emerged. I could not have conspired such a bizarre way of returning to my Soul, my union with God, and to live as my authentic self.

What is your particular story that will, through your own deliberate intention, invite you to see and experience your life in a totally new way? Don't wallow in your anguish for eternity. Don't waste your distress; let it become your most profound gift that leads you to find yourself in the center of the stone.

Healing our stories brings us to our deepest longings. Know that it is possible for you, an ordinary person, to live a passionate life that is anything but ordinary. Understand that your contributions to the world are necessary and give them freely, without need for recognition or special dispensation. Honor the mystery of yourself. Be willing to tolerate your imperfections as well as the consequences of your magnificence. Your past, while it influences your future, does not dictate it. Nurture and honor the glory within you that is your birthright. Allow the healing of your stories to lead you to find your true name.

*"And the day came when the risk to remain tight in a bud
was more painful than the risk it took to blossom."*

Anaïs Nin

"It is never too late to be who you might have been."

George Elliott

*"Great acting is being able to create a character.
Great character is being able to be yourself."*

John Leguizamo

*"It is important from time to time to slow down,
to go away by yourself, and simply BE."*

Eileen Cadd

*"Yesterday I was clever, so I decided to change the world.
Today I am wise, so I decided to change myself instead."*

-Rumi

Chapter Ten

IT TAKES A LIFETIME

OCTOBER, 1996

B RENT AND I ARE IN AN EVENING STUDY GROUP AT CHURCH. WE are in class to learn, but more than that, we want to be near the new pastor, Reverend Ken Williamson. He is an intense, raw, deeply passionate human who speaks truth from his soul. I like him and I believe his authentic way of teaching. I might even say I trust him a little. He's discussing the concept of prayer being answered.

I have an immediate negative reaction. I seethe with fury and am filled with mourning once again. God is a mocking, malevolent trickster. He's a hoax, no more real than the wizard from Oz.

Reverend Ken responds to my outburst of pain. He begins speaking to me about "healers." I'm baffled. A woman sitting beside me calmly takes my hand and says, "Shelli, there are healers in this world; I'm one of them."

With complete sincerity I ask, "What is a healer?" I have absolutely no idea what she means. I question her. "Does that mean you have special powers?" Inside I think, *How could I not have known that someone right in this room can restore my vision? And if it is so, by God, I want her to do it right this minute.*

The fantasy about healing that I created was not, however, what I would eventually learn healing was all about.

I studied the art and science of energy medicine, personal and trans-personal psychology for eight years. But those eight years of formal education are not what makes me the healer I am today. Socrates said, "In an instant a life may turn around, a heart may open in a moment of grace, a body may be healed. But preparing for that moment can take a lifetime...."

Every event of my entire life has been necessary to lead me to my own healing and my work as a healer, which is the case for all of us. It is unfortunate when people are not able to recognize the healing nestled in the stories of their lives. Hopefully, you are finding that every story in your life leads to a blessing of renewal. In my work with students and clients I often say, "I needed every bit of pain I experienced to realize I didn't need to hurt all the time."

MY CHILDHOOD

As a child in the early years, I had no awareness of the concept of The Divine or the truth that God and I are one. My spiritual experience was limited to church with a girlfriend at a strict and punitive institution. Here I learned to fear God, an entity whom I didn't know and didn't want to know based on what I was being taught. My family proclaimed to be Protestant Christians, a term I learned by hearing Mom use it as I was once being admitted to the hospital. We celebrated the traditional Christian holidays of Christmas and Easter, but we never attended weekly church services as a family. Although raised with church as a center stone of his youth, my dad is a publicly proclaimed agnostic; he believes in nothing beyond what he can see and feel. Never was there any talk about finding healing through anything other than the doctor's office and a prescription.

No one prayed or mentioned prayer. I learned that anything I received I acquired through my own efforts. This helped me form a distorted belief system that said life is competitive instead of companionable. This belief germinated yet another distortion: a belief that I am alone in an uncaring world. I did not believe that the universe, God, was supportive, especially of me. I knew I'd better be willful, strong, and self-reliant if I wanted to survive in what I felt was a hostile, cut-throat world.

MY ADOLESCENCE

As I reached adolescence, about the time I was diagnosed with diabetes, I began to see non-human entities. Later in life I realized they were appearing for two distinct reasons: to help me cope with diabetes and my emotional struggles at the time, and to dispel my misconception about a supportive universal force. Instead of providing comfort or strength, seeing the entities froze me in terror.

I'm awakened in the lonely hours after midnight. I'm drowsy, but I'm being pulled to sit up, wake up. The light in my bedroom is dim. The glow of the streetlight allows me to see my doll sitting on the chair, the bookshelves on the wall that are lined with my important possessions, and the door to the hallway which is just eight feet away.

My gaze centers on the doorway and I see her standing there, again, the ghostly appearing woman. She looks the same as always, dressed in a long, white, flowing dress. She carries flowers in her left hand. Her face gives no clue of her mood but she looks directly at me, just like she always does. I'm terrified. I want to scream. I want Dad to wake up and get her out of my room, but my voice doesn't work.

Now she walks into the room, slowly strolling back and forth in front of my bed as I watch her, panic-stricken. She stops, looks at me again, and I scoot away as best I can on my narrow bed and flatten my back against the wall. As I do, she dissolves into the darkness. She'll be back again, I know, maybe not for several months or even a year, but she, or one of the others, will come back.

These entities appeared as living people. I didn't recognize any of them when I was a child. I still remember some of their exact features today. They woke me up at night and appeared to me. One was the woman with the long, flowing white dress. Another woman had very long, dark hair, tanned skin, and primitive clothes. There were a couple of men whose images aren't as vivid in my memory, but one man who stands out was clad in a double-breasted coat, had a narrow face and brown eyes, and wore a fedora-like hat.

I knew they wanted to communicate with me, but I was too afraid to speak to them. I was equally afraid to mention the visits to my parents or friends, afraid they would poke fun at me or tell me it was just a dream. Eventually the spirits appeared during the daytime. I didn't like this at all! When it happened I was always alone. I looked directly at them; they acknowledged me, but I was mute with terror. In time, they stopped showing up. In retrospect, I think they left because they knew they were frightening me.

MY BLINDNESS

Being a healer initially took on a traditional role. I thrived in science and biology. In addition to the various medical events in this book, I was hospitalized every year of my life from the time I was eighteen months old. My mom worked in a hospital. Hospitals felt like home to me. My own medical conditions fostered my fascination with medicine and healing. I became a Registered Nurse. I loved the Emergency Department where I worked during college and for a time before I married Tom. Deep physical trauma didn't scare me. Being a part of saving lives was a satisfying feeling. I discovered I also loved being present for the family members who were also in crisis, and I was good at it. In college, psychology classes were easy and interesting. I discovered I liked sorting out my own emotional turmoil, but assisting others was something I found profoundly gratifying. People had always come to me with problems, needing a compassionate ear or sound advice.

When, at twenty-three, I began losing my sight in Holland, I was overwrought with grief. In the exhaustion of kidney failure, there was no opportunity to witness any healing moments. I realized I had to have something other than myself to support me; I couldn't do it on my own. This was clear. So I decided to try out this God idea, and I began praying and considering whether God could be real.

Once Scott gave me his kidney and my health instantly improved, I was able to look back on my two years of kidney failure and newly acquired blindness. I began seeing how healing might spring from those events. I knew my life would be whatever I made it. I was hopeful this "god" whom I didn't know well at all would begin to materialize. But I still held a belief that I had to do the heavy work on my own. Although still hesitant and reserved about my trust in God, I prayed often in gratitude. I was beginning to understand that despite my circumstances, I was, and always would be okay, yet I couldn't justify my belief at this time. I just knew that I knew.

After I lost my sight, the spiritual entities returned with more vigor than when I was a child. I first feel the spiritual entities near me. It feels exactly like a real human standing very close to me. Back then, it scared the hell out of me just as it did when I was a child. I might be in the laundry room or standing at the bathroom vanity, any place where my back is open to the room.

I feel a presence over my left shoulder and back and extending above my head. Shocked, I gasp and spin around believing an intruder has entered my house. I can see it very distinctly. I'm disturbed because I'm not supposed to see anything. Yet the image is distinct, the sensation vivid. There is someone suspended at my back. I quickly reach out defensively; whoever it is must be there to hurt me. But when I reach, my arm pushes through air. There is no material person standing there.

I feel a bit crazy, but I know what I'm feeling. I know that I'm seeing what I see, but how can this be? I can't tell Tom; he'd be very upset. When I told him what had happened the day the beast came up our stairway, he was furious, believing I was either insane or conjuring up the entire ordeal. So I keep my secret again.

Sometimes I walk through a space of the house and I feel them as I pass by. My fear of them haunts me. Soon I become afraid to stay in our home alone. Flash backs of the devilish beast resurface. Although I knew something was in the room with me, I couldn't differentiate whether it was a menacing threat, either spiritual or living, or a peaceful Being of Light. The sensation I experienced with the spirits felt exactly the same as when a live person came close to me. Because I didn't understand, I decided they were threatening. I wanted them to go away, and they did, for a while.

BEGINNING THE PATH TO HEALER

Once I was separated from Tom, I was free to choose my own belief system. I was introduced to Rumi, the great Sufi mystic and his poetry, and I was catapulted into a realm where I instantly felt at home. I was instinctively drawn to my spiritual nature, my communion with all things holy, and to God. Once released from the imposed viewpoints of others, I easily assumed my true nature as a sacred being who, although still ordinary, knows the truth about healing and the holiness within all people.

The spiritual entities returned, but now I was not afraid. I began to listen to the messages I was receiving from the Divine, starting to discern wisdom from fantasy. I began to find purpose and deeper meaning in the circumstances of my life, and considered the possibility of a loving God. I was beginning to find my true self.

I became inspired by my discontentment. In my personal and professional life I've seen traditional medicine work many times, but fail too often. I was eager to find ways to help myself and others to live a healthier and more fulfilled life. I began a course of study and became a certified hypnotherapist. I realized that I had successfully incorporated blindness, diabetes, and a kidney transplant into my life by focused intention, which is the foundation of hypnotherapy. This, along with taking college writing courses where I learned to express my emotions, pacified me for a while.

BRENT, MY TEACHER AND KIND TRUE LOVE

Brent came into my life and allowed me to delve more deeply into a world that my nuclear family, and Tom, would have mocked. I tell him about my experiences perceiving spirits. Even though I'm not afraid of them now, I think it's fringy and bizarre. But Brent thinks it's normal. I explain my passion to understand God as more than a concept. He is years ahead of me. Often times Brent discusses deep spiritual theories with me in what I call, "Green Eggs and Ham" mentality. Instead of being complex and philosophical, using extraneous, esoteric words, he's pure and simple, and he makes total sense.

As I began my reading and studies of energy medicine and psychological transformation that includes the spiritual side of being human, it is Brent who kept me grounded with his no-nonsense explanations. When I first began to hear the voice of God, I thought it was abnormal, even weird and something I "shouldn't be doing." Brent kept me calm.

I didn't understand this ability, but Brent saw it as a normal part of life. "People do this all the time; they just don't know they're doing it. They probably call it something else. Do you think people conversed with God during Biblical times and then it suddenly stopped?" he asked in his calm, confident manner.

MY FORMAL HEALING EDUCATION

Three years after the evening in church with Reverend Ken I began my formal studies in energy medicine healing. I arrived at school in 1999 with no more knowledge about healing or being a healer than I had back at church. I couldn't explain what I was studying to others; I didn't know myself. I had never read a book on energy medicine and had never heard the word "chakra." I simply knew I was supposed to go.

I despised the entire experience at first. Even as I finished my sixth year and was in teacher training, I often hated it. Each time Brent drove me to the airport to fly to school I said the same thing, "I think I'll stay home." It was hard and often times a lonely experience. Parts of me thought I was being irresponsible and ridiculous. I had substantial issues that were not ordinary. I'm flying every other month unescorted across the country: blind, with brittle diabetes, seven stents in my heart, and a kidney transplant that was barely working during the last two years of my travel.

I was exceedingly tense and fearful. I was afraid of the people, my limitations, and my special needs that others would be asked to meet, and I was even afraid I'd die. A man drowned at school during my first year and my fears about dying grew exponentially. Then the terrorist attack of 9/11. Boarding a plane two weeks later, I felt my heart race and anxiety flutter in my stomach. Yet despite my fears, my confidence and healing abilities continued to develop.

At first I was afraid I couldn't do the healing skills because I couldn't watch the demonstrations. But to my amazement, the skills were already within me! I believed I wouldn't understand the science because many of the books weren't audio recorded for me. Again, I was fascinated that I understood complex concepts from an innate knowing. I honestly never "learned" a skill; I became the skill. Laying my hands on another student to do practice healings was my sanctuary while at school. I could touch, so I could "see."

As students, we were also learning to be more authentic. Sometimes this included people letting me know my blindness and special needs made them angry. Sometimes it meant people telling me they hated me or were jealous of my ability to see beyond the physical. Sometimes it meant people telling me how much they loved me. It was all equally difficult to hear. The six years of study tore me open. And it put me together with a stronger foundation on which to build.

To say I was naive at first would be an extreme understatement. Since the theme of the first year was "Healing the self" I believed that blindness, kidney failure, and diabetes would be wiped out before the year elapsed! When it became apparent that this was not the case, I was livid. *What sort of healing of the self is going to happen if we aren't to be rid of desperate diseases and conditions?* I asked.

I entered school carrying a combative belief system, a foundational theory that life is a battlefield. I believed mistrust was essential for survival. Beneath the mistrust lay my fear that I would be betrayed, again. Even my closest friend, parents, allies could betray me. My own body had already failed me. I was split between trusting and mistrusting God. I wanted to trust, but what reason did I have for doing so? After all, I had been to many altar calls for healings. None of the thousands of prayers said on my behalf saved my eyesight. Mom had a plaque on the wall of our kitchen when I was growing up. It read, "God answers prayers." After I lost my sight, I made her take it down.

I began my education as a healer at odds with God and with anyone who gave me the slightest inkling that they might deceive me. Holding God, and everyone at arm's length felt lonely, but less dangerous than the risk of being betrayed.

Have you ever held back on beginning a new idea or embarking on a new journey because you thought you might look foolish or that it was impractical? Despite your lack of prior exposure or understanding you can go into the world and learn new things. You don't need to leave behind your entire self-identity to do so. In fact, as you take the risk to discover and nurture latent aspirations, you could very well unearth pieces of yourself you didn't even know were there.

Many of us are unsettled, restless, and know there is something in the center of our being that aches to be discovered, something we wish to learn or to do. I waited to start this book, making all sorts of excuses as to why writing a book was impossible and impractical. When I definitively started writing, all of the excuses I had created dissolved. My intention to finally do what I had longed to do signaled the universe. People appeared who helped me birth my creation. Tongue-in-cheek, I call them my doulas. The same sort of thing can happen for you when you deliberately make up your mind and take your first steps toward what it is you've always wanted to do.

The desire to follow our dreams does not emerge from our rational minds. It arises from a sense that often is tangential to reason and logic. Sometimes we have no explanation for our longings other than a feeling that if we don't act, something important inside will perish. People who are committed to their reason believe that following an unexplainable dream is dangerous and silly. Reason-oriented people will try to convince us we are being irrational, and we are. Desires of the soul and heart aren't rational, they're intuitive, which is emotionally driven. So long as we aren't expecting someone else to finance our dreams (or bail us out if they fail), and we aren't imposing our impulse onto unwilling participants, we ought to learn new things and begin new journeys, even if they seem wild.

In the beginning of my education, I could find little value in emotional healing. I wanted physical resolution or nothing. The only way I was going to make peace with God was if He (always seen as masculine back then) started giving me all the promises forecasted for me in the Bible. I was setting God up to fail. If He couldn't eradicate my blindness and diabetes, it was proof that He was a liar and a fraud. As long as He proved to be a phony, I could hold on to my mistrust and anger.

I was attached to the negative pleasure derived from victim-consciousness. In my injured, hostile place, I loved that no one could help me with my problems. In this state, I was unapproachable. I shot down any suggestion of possible healing before my companion or teacher had an idea out of their mouths. I pushed everyone and everything down with my negativity and aggression. If I couldn't have the healing I demanded, I refused to engage. Down deep, some part of me loved feeling my hostile power and control.

In time, I grew weary of this coping strategy. I was using a lot of energy to keep myself separate, hold my pain in place, and dismiss the authentic help that others and the universe were offering me. And doing so prevented me from recognizing the joy that was mine for the taking.

I came to realize that this was not about me trusting God. What I'd wanted was a guarantee that I wouldn't have to suffer any more. Without this guarantee, I felt lost, unsafe, and prone to horrible occurrences I didn't believe I had the capacity to manage. So my healing moment was seeing that it wasn't about me trusting God, but trusting me to be strong or wise enough to cope with whatever might come my way. Not God's lack of strength, but mine. This realization was the impetus for me to change my beliefs about God. Once I saw that I didn't hate or fear God, but rather I'd feared the unpredictability of life, I was able to shift my focus to me rather than on Him.

Next, I confronted my attachment to seeing God as masculine.

My mistrust of the masculine God was largely based on a lifetime of experiences that left me feeling betrayed by men, especially those closest to me. I realized that I needed to change my image of God from masculine to feminine in order for me to develop trust in the Divine, and later I let go of any gendered image of the Creator.

My teacher affirmed my ability to see and feel beyond our normal senses. This helped to tame my embarrassment and insecurity about my real life experiences. Many of my close friends, co-workers and family, thought I had gone off the deep end or was making it all up. Because I was irreverent, people thought I was joking when I talked about being a spiritual healer and therapist. "Spiritual people don't curse. They certainly don't have anger or judgmental thoughts," I often heard.

One of my dearest friends took me aside and quoted Biblical Scripture, saying I would go to hell for pursuing this type of work. Her words didn't help me feel safe. What I needed at that time was to embrace a God that wasn't punitive, demanding of obedience, or promising love only if certain conditions were met. The God my friend pointed out to me through the Scriptures reminded me of the cold, heartless God in the church of my girlfriend during my youth. That God reminded me of authority figures in my life, whose ruling nature intimidated and scared me. I doubted I could meet their expectations. How would I ever meet the requirements of the God described to me by my friend?

My friend's words, while confusing and frightening at first, actually encouraged me to explore, consider and define who God actually was to me. I simply couldn't abide a God who wasn't all-loving, always, to all people. I realize that some people choose their religion, but ninety percent of the world are born into their faiths. I self-identify as a Christian because I was born into it. Had I been born in Pakistan, I suppose I would have self-identified as a Buddhist or Muslim for the same reason. The idea that my soul would go to hell based on my human choices was ridiculous to me. My soul didn't have thoughts, opinions, or beliefs. It didn't make choices; my human brain did. The more I trusted that the energy of God was my ally in this work, the more I trusted my abilities to perceive. Seeing, feeling, and knowing beyond what is evident became extremely natural for me.

LESSONS FROM MY KIDNEY-PANCREAS TRANSPLANT

When it was time for me to have the kidney pancreas transplant, I had been working as a therapist and energy medicine professional for some time. I understood the need to accept the parts of my body that weren't actually mine. I used my ability to align my intention, my kavanah, to allow Spirit to bring me the perfect organs for my body. I embraced my newfound belief in unity and companionship rather than my old belief that life is competitive and divisive. I believe this shift of consciousness permitted my body to receive the organs with ease and graceful elegance.

The double organ transplant taught me how to receive graciously and with humility. Giving had always been easy for me, but receiving implies vulnerability. Receiving meant I had to admit I had needs. My fear had always been that those needs wouldn't be met, so I denied having them. I worked hard to soften my fear of vulnerability and all the beliefs I held about what could happen to me if I were vulnerable. I was able to admit that receiving was an acceptable and necessary transaction. Each day I deliberately worked to open my throat and heart to take in the love people sent to me during my surgery and recovery, including the beautiful gift from my kidney donor, Jason and his family, and the family of my pancreas donor. I observed the wisdom of nature often, looking at how the organic universe thrives with its perfect balance of giving and receiving, the yin and yang.

When I was diagnosed with the first pancreas rejection and parallel kidney cancer, I was thrown off-guard. Everything had been working so well, so unencumbered. After recovering from the reeling thought that I could either die from malignant kidney cancer or lose the pancreas and return to life with diabetes, I searched for the most useful way to address the final stressor present at that time: my kidney donor's emotions. I observed the two sides of me, the injured, young side and the recovered, mature side as they wrestled to be the louder voice.

My Higher Self, the more healed side of me, knew I had to prioritize me before addressing Jason's emotions. Once my health stabilized, I had more clarity and reserve to try to resolve the conflict that had arisen between us. I understood that we all want our experiences validated. As I allowed my compassion to Jason's dilemma to lead my actions, healing for each of us emerged.

MY LESSONS FROM LYMPHOMA

Being diagnosed with lymphoma moved me from a place of experiencing the Divine to a place of being "Source Embodied," a term I've adopted from a colleague and friend, Dan Cohen, MD, who's dedicated his life to understanding his spiritual nature. Although my entire life has been a struggle to stay alive, the enormity of a systemic cancer was a threat to my life in a way much different than prior situations. Lymphoma gave me the opportunity to solidly choose full living, despite my current limitations and regardless of what the future would hold. My spiritual development was again put to the test. Would I trust in a loving God despite another catastrophic illness, or would I throw in the towel and decide I had been right after all: God is a hoax?

My process as a Healer allowed me my initial calm acceptance that death may be the outcome this time. My spiritual healing allowed me to look at death from two sides, the side of me that could survive and the side that could expire. I'm not suggesting that I'd surrendered to my death without periods of struggle and fear, but I was able to find true peace and a sense of safety between moments of insecurity while awaiting my final diagnosis and prognosis. In due time, I moved to an unyielding desire to live. Yet during my treatment course, and even afterward, I considered the possibility of my imminent death and what it meant.

When a person is diagnosed with cancer, especially a systemic cancer, mortality becomes very real. Here I had been coping with life and death situations for years, but now it seemed the idea that I could die, really die, was no longer an intellectual concept. I could feel my death nearly touching me. *How can the world go on without me?* my ego asked. *One day I will become worm food, simple dust. In less than a generation, no one will remember me or anything I've done or said.* This was my human response to lymphoma.

The spiritual side of me understood the entire process of lymphoma: diagnosis, treatment, side effects and anything else it brought, would provide a transfiguration, a particular wisdom for my soul that I had not yet developed. If I should die from this illness, I knew it wouldn't be only the end of my life, rather, the beginning of another. I trusted that if I should die, a brilliant love would be waiting, eager to receive me. I would be with all the spiritual entities I have been with here in the physical dimension for many decades already. Some theologians believe the journey of death is traveled alone. I believe a heavenly host of souls will gather me up and carry me effortlessly with them.

Within that belief, death doesn't terrify me. Unlike past situations wherein I was furious that I had to endure yet another monumental medical ailment, I instead accepted the situation for what I believed it to be, an opportunity to feel myself unified with God and to be faithful in my faith in an even more steadfast way.

Beyond my thoughts of mortality and soul growth, I wanted the cancer to be cured. It was a deliberate choice rather than a hope. I knew that every single moment of wounding and healing I'd experienced in my lifetime was necessary to help me embrace myself as "Source."

I was able to hold the cancer in my body differently than I had done with previous conditions. In the case of diabetes so long ago, I reached a point of partial acceptance, by seeing the illness as an entity with consciousness. What was different in the case of lymphoma was that I not only saw the cancer as a live entity, but also as something I needed to love instead of hate. It wasn't easy, but I knew it was necessary. Being aggressive and oppositional creates disharmony in me. It creates tension and stress in my mind and body. It makes me lose my faith. I didn't want to feel that way. And I couldn't imagine that it would serve me in reaching a cure. Focusing on love makes me feel vital, safe, and calm. Love is the true aspect of the soul, the state of being from which I try to live each day.

The bigger idea here is that I chose Love over hatred, fear, and desperation. Maybe that didn't do anything to cure the cancer, but it taught me that even in a tragic situation I have the power to choose. Lymphoma helped me to start to adopt the ability to choose Love regardless of the outcome. I used to think it was my will that got things done and kept me safe. But I know now that Love is the creative force in the universe. It is Love that heals everything. It's not that Love alone could cure the lymphoma, although a part of me knows that Love is the healing force that cures everything, but that Love certainly heals *me*, whether I live or die. And that's the true salvation, the healing: being able to lean on Love, trust Love, believe in Love, and *be* Love.

My journey as a Healer continues daily. The moment I believe "I've arrived, I'm all done!" is the day I know I surely have much further to go. I seek grace daily. My healing abilities grow with my times of weakness and strife. They take me another step beyond my imagined limitations and closer to God. I welcome in "the uninvited guest," as Rumi calls it. It's the thing that appears to be what we don't want. I know the uninvited guest, if I allow it, will help me to be more of who I truly am.

One of my teachers once told me "You are a profound healer, and it's because of your profound wounding." At the time, I was only beginning to accept the truth of this statement. I have a better grasp today of what that means. I don't hope for more catastrophic occurrences, rather, I ask for easy troubles that help me grow and appreciate my blessings.

As a nurse in the emergency room, I helped to save lives. As a healer, I'm helping to change them. In the long run, a life saved is beautiful and lasts for the moment, but a life changed is miraculous and lasts into eternity.

And so it is.

Sometimes we hesitate to begin our healing. Sometimes our reluctance is our fear of changing. Sometimes we're even afraid to let go of the pain, because if we no longer have the pain, we believe the truth of our experience will no longer be valid, that it wasn't as reprehensible as it truly was. We think that people will only see the healed, happy person, and won't appreciate the enormous effort we've invested in repairing our lives. Worse yet, we fear we will use up all the healing forces available, and we will feel no better than we did before we started. We fear changing a system that, although imperfect, is at least getting us through each day. We believe it's not the right time, or the conditions aren't right, or a flurry of other excuses. There is no perfect time to begin to heal, but for certain, the right time is when we are broken, not when we are all put together.

We are all wounded. We are all afraid. If we were honest, we would all admit that we fear our weakness and insecurity in many areas of our lives. We all share a common wish that holds us together as people committed to our own healing; to blaze a trail that leads us to our authentic selves. First we become naked, stripped of all the ways we've hidden our true nature. The truth is, our false self and our limiting beliefs must die, the part of us that feels stupid, fragile, incapable, and idiotic.

When this part falls away, the truth is that we are not dying, we are beginning to live.

THE HEALING

All of my life experiences have been sequential learnings that have guided me to my unique ministry as a healer. Every event, including those not mentioned in this book, have shored up my ability to walk through life with much more confidence. This confidence translates to more solidity of presence. This presence is not the presence of my ego-based identity where I hunger for the approval of others before I can feel safe, or frantically search for right answers or impose my beliefs onto the group. I'm able to maintain my true presence as someone who is continuously paying attention to these normal ego insecurities so that I, and people I'm with, can feel the presence of my soul.

My true soul qualities still have unique personality quirks and characteristics. I'm still sarcastic and funny. I'm still determined and passionate. As I became aware of who I was not, I became more authentically who I am, and was willing to be this, openly.

The ideas I formed about God in my younger years have evolved. Today I have a maturing concept about God and the nature of God. I've even changed much of the language I use to refer to God, now using terms I feel more fitting for this universal, ubiquitous energy, names such as The Divine, Source, The Creator, and yes, God. As I broadened my understanding about who I am, I also expanded my understanding about who, and what, God is.

My unfolding appreciation of God healed most of my early feelings of betrayal and abandonment. I'm now able to rest more fully in an abiding faith. My soulful prayers are now a communion with God rather than *me* asking for some favor. Instead, I commune with God as my brother, sister, compassionate healer. I call on Jesus and His Christ presence because I'm a Christian and that's my way, but it's not the only way. As Rumi said, "Christians do Christian things, Hindus do Hindu things. What difference does it make? An ocean diver doesn't need snowshoes." My prayers are affirming rather than beseeching.

In the past I wanted proof of God's existence. I wanted a sign, a demonstration of His or Her presence in my life. I'd been waiting for an epiphany and all the while missing God's presence. I learned that God is everywhere; there is no place God is not. Before my journey to healing and becoming a healer, I could not have been convinced of this truth. All of my difficult experiences, laced with the miraculous healings of those experiences, taught me about the mystery of God.

To know God I needed to stop searching outside myself and start looking within. Only here would I be able to experience God. Now I watch spring burst through the cool soil of the earth and witness God. I listen to birds of every kind in the trees sing the name of God. I experience another's sorrow or exuberance and feel God. Recognizing God in these everyday happenings is the epiphany.

Realizing that God is within me and that I am in God changed my entire perspective on the journey of my life and is a cornerstone of my work as a professional healer. Today I can feel the eternal presence of The Divine within my thoughts and most importantly, in my body.

As I traversed the many stages of my life-long journey to becoming a healer, I first believed my seemingly broken body could not possibly be a temple of The Divine. As I grew into myself as a Healer, my beliefs about the condition of my body changed. No longer did I consider my physical ailments as brokenness, but instead, as opportunities for the grace of God to work through me. The magnificence of God is not found in the perfection of things, but rather, in the perfect imperfection.

Instead of my willful insistence that my body be healed in my timing and in the manner I previously demanded, I'm now more able to allow the Divine timing of the universe to unfold. It's so much easier, so much simpler! Things my ego thought were critical, I've learned are much less so.

My healing virtues and abilities emerged instinctively. I became cognizant of what had always been within me as I discarded all of the prior ways I stayed small, demanded to be important, remained hidden or conversely, burst into rooms. I healed the limiting parts of my stories. Underneath the sludge of pain was a pulsing embryo waiting to be born. The embryo was the aspect of God inside me, which contained all of who I am and my potential, including my Glory and my healing abilities. I came to fully realize that the healing that comes through me is not a talent or technique. Rather, the healing lies in my ability to forego my ego thoughts and beliefs and become the energy of God that pulses through me, and everyone. The skill I'm learning to hone, if it can be called that, is the ability to maintain a pure intention to allow Rukha d' Koodsha to effortlessly move through me. The literal translation of "Rukha d'Koodsha" is "Spirit of the Holy," or, in commonly understood terms, Holy Spirit.

This Holiness is not associated with any religion or doctrine. It is the energy that created, and continues to create, the entire universe. Names are meaningless to this energy. Words cannot label its grace and being, because it existed before terms and language were devised. It is the eternal energy that has no shape or designation, no form or thought other than unconditional love.

I learned the power of vulnerability. Brené Brown's inspiring Ted Talk confirmed what I already knew; vulnerability is not a weakness, it is a strength. It was through my struggle, my mistakes, and re-starts in understanding who I was, and who I was not as a healer that I learned that all birth is painful and hesitant.

Before I could guide others on their own passage to their healing, I needed to travel my own path. I could only be a light for someone else when I had illuminated my own darkness. Stepping into that darkness went against every instinct in my body. I felt intimidated and exposed in my vulnerability. If I wanted to be the person I'd always wanted to be, I could not run from the risk of looking like a fool or being criticized by the nay-sayers, and there were plenty of those. I needed to risk the possibility of failing ten times in order to be successful only once. I had to be willing to turn my beliefs, mostly about myself, upside-down. To be the effective healer I wanted to be I had to change, and to change, I needed to be vulnerable. I learned that being vulnerable is my most natural state. I spent the first half of my life trying to avoid it. I'm spending the second half returning to it.

I honor every event in my life as useful to show me how to live as my Light and not as my misfortune. Embracing my difficulties, my trauma, and all of my mistakes and poor judgments, I allow shame and embarrassment to be replaced with a sense of compunction. Rather than judgment, this is a regret. When I move into a state of compunction rather than self-loathing or ruminating on my errors, I can more easily offer self-forgiveness, which is much more satisfying than being forgiven.

The art of my work is dependent on the times I fumble. Without these times I would have no grist for the mill, so to speak. I would have no fuel for the fire, no incentive to strive to improve myself and my art, and thus fulfill my mission not only as a healer but as a Soul-driven person who enjoys a fulfilling life regardless of circumstance.

Every moment is sacred and hallowed. Every story blessed with opportunity for healing and a more fulfilled life. I am in Source and Source is in me. When I allow this belief to prevail, I'm able to relax long enough to allow my crazy thinking, the thinking that tries to convince me I'm a shameful mess and unworthy of brilliance, to be quieted. The more my actions, thoughts, and beliefs spring from my faith in my innate goodness, the more my tiresome thoughts that keep me bound in chains and playing small melt away. I experience freedom and I'm able to know my place in the world. Then, and only then, I become the healer the world needs.

All of us are healers in our own right. The healer within you emerges as a cheerful waitress, a humorous technician, a compassionate architect, and a friend who listens with sensitivity. We each have the potential to be a peacemaker and a Samaritan. Any one of us is a life-saver as an organ donor or a blood donor. We are a change maker when we graciously give of our time and talents.

No matter what our job is in life, all functions are sacred. Everyone has the opportunity to be a worker of miracles as an ordinary person. Retirees are the sages and the holy volunteers. Mothers and fathers are nurturing the next generation of heroes and heroines. You can influence the health of your communities by going about your day and your work with conscious intention to share your in-born healing abilities that naturally emanate from your heart. Many people who attend formal education in energy healing never open a private practice. These people apply their learning in the boardrooms and offices where they work as computer programmers and stock brokers.

We all become healers when we stop seeing our jobs simply as a way to earn money. When we look outside ourselves and recognize that we can change the energy of our workplace, we become healers. We can purposely decide to be the employee who is supportive of teammates. We can be the person everyone looks forward to working with because of our positivity instead of being the one who everyone avoids because of complaining and gossip.

What are your ordained gifts and honorable qualities that can make a difference in your home, neighborhood, your city or your place of work? You might think you don't have much to offer because you're just an ordinary person. We may not be famous, but each of us can be an important healer in someone's life.

To know what your intrinsic gifts are, simply look at the characteristics and skills that are inherent strengths. In general, they will be attributes that you are known for. You could be inherently orderly, funny, or a great communicator.

Do something on a regular basis that comes from your heart-centered soul. Avoid looking for something grand to do. This is a set-up for failure because you've chosen a task that's unsustainable. Rather, do a little thing and offer it consistently. Don't give from obligation or for hopes of acknowledgement. Instead, do it because it makes your heart and soul happy. Every event in our lives has served as our own healing and has sculpted us into the healers we are now. What events in your life have revealed your previously unrealized talents and assets? In a world that would rather punish the self or ostracize the misdirected, it's essential we accept and honor our mistakes as growth opportunities that open us to our healing virtues. Use your acquired wisdom to be a healing light for others.

Be bold, be brave, and dare to claim and share your necessary and intrinsic worth. As you walk through life, decide to leave a footprint of love on every doorstep. When you touch a single life, your small gesture becomes great because when one amongst us is served, many are affected.

"The gift you carry for others is not an attempt to save the world but to belong to it. It's not possible to save the world by trying to save it. You need to find what is genuinely yours to offer the world before you can make it a better place. Discovering your unique gifts to bring to your community is your greatest opportunity and challenge. That offering of that gift – your true self – is the most you can do to love and serve the world. And it's all the world needs."

Joseph Campbell

"I repose in myself. And that part of myself, that deepest and richest part in which I repose, is what I call 'God.'"

Etty Hillesum

AFTERWORD

Today I sat pensively on the cool cobblestone steps in front of our house. It is late in the afternoon on a warm October day; the last of the sunshine dappled through the colored leaves on the branches of the trees. I remembered how many similar hours I spent sitting on the steps of my parents' home. I was in one of those "moods," just like back then. The dried seeds from our flower garden and already fallen leaves blew restfully around me. I felt the eternalness of the sun on my face. And I wondered: *Am I foolish to believe? Am I alone? Is there truly a God who hears my every thought? Are there really spiritual helpers surrounding me that listen to my voice?*

In the distance I heard a neighbor raking, further off the sound of geese migrating. I wondered what it was like for the geese to see the earth from above. I wondered what it felt like for the creatures under the crust of the soil, having the earth cool and the rake scraping across their ceiling. I was swept up in my contemplative and ever-present curiosity about the mystery of the universe.

There I sat, my arms on my knees just like I did forty years ago. I felt a whisper of security return as I realized I was still the "Me" I have always been even though I've changed. I felt momentary reassurance that the universe remained constant in its enigmatic mysteriousness. And yet, the mystery also felt ominous, too pervasive, and I questioned my past experiences with Source. I longed for confirmation. A tear slid down my cheek. This day I felt like the world was empty, and so was heaven. Why, I don't honestly know. Even the geese and the neighbor seemed unreachable.

Just because I've been able to extract healings and blessings from the trials of my life doesn't mean I don't have times of doubt or dread about the current moment or about my future. Just because I can feel myself as a Divine being, doesn't mean I'm always able to sit in the lap of tranquility. I can fall into an invisible hole, suddenly feeling misty, alone, or scared on a simple, ordinary day.

I spoke aloud to the mild October air. "Please show me you're really here. Help me remember the times I've felt you close. I'm calling you, angels. Don't forget me. Don't leave me." I waited, hoped, reached with all my being to find the reassuring signal I so needed. Nothing.

I remembered walking through the cemetery one Memorial Day with Aunt Donna. Donna and I are walking along the gravel roadway in the cemetery, heading for my grandparents' graves. I distinctly heard feet rustling through tall grass beside us, but when I asked Donna who it was, she said there was no one there. When we stopped walking so I could focus on what I was sensing and hearing, the sound of shuffling feet and rustling grass stopped. We took two steps; the invisible feet took two steps. We waited; it waited. We continued on; the unseen companion followed steadily at our side.

Pointing toward the sound I asked Donna, "Who is walking there?" Looking around she said with puzzlement, "No one, Shelli."

"There must be. Can't you hear the footsteps through the tall grass?" I heard it as clearly as Donna's voice and the birds in the trees. "It's right here, here, in this tall grass." I stepped off the gravel roadway and found nothing other than trimmed lawn. I say aloud, "Okay, I know you're there. I hear you. Just come along with us." And the sound of the feet walking through tall grass stayed with us for the rest of the afternoon as we visited our family's burial sites.

Recalling the experience now as I sat on the steps I said, "Okay, that was real."

My mind jumped to the night on Cape Hatteras when my "spirit chain" showed up. My friend Tim and I were vacationing in early November of 1995. We rent a mobile home on the beach of the craggy shoreline where Blue Beard and other prates of his day hid out. That night, before Tim and I go to sleep, I am distressed. I'd forgotten my Medic-Alert necklace at home, the one that says I have diabetes. I mention my anxiety about traveling without it several times before finally resigning myself to let it go.

Now it is the middle of the night. I am sleeping alone in the bedroom at one end of the mobile home when I awake. A horrific storm is raging. Ferocious winds blow off the ocean water. The home shakes and rumbles on its foundation. As I lay in the bed, listening with amazement to the thrilling ocean storm, I wonder, *How is this little trailer staying moored?*

To my astonishment, I hear voices shout, and heavy chains rattle outside the window facing the beach-front. I'm mystified. This storm is way too intense for people to be out in it. I lay motionless listening to the activity on the beach. I wish I could look out the window. As I strain to get a sense of what is happening outside, an unmistakable, enormous energy moves around the side of the house. It deliberately turns the corner and comes to rest, hovering outside the window behind the head of my bed. I am both intensely curious and a bit scared. My curiosity vanishes when the sound of a chain jangles inches from my head.

I shout above the howling wind, "Tim! Tim! Get in here!" He can't hear me above the violent storm. The massive energy outside the window feels scintillating against my skin. Instantly, I feel its massiveness stretching high above the roof-line. The sound of the chain continues while the wind howls and the trailer rocks.

Finally, Tim hears my cries for help. He walks into the bedroom and as he crosses the threshold, poof! Everything becomes silent and still. The energy evaporates.

In the morning I find draped over the headboard of the bed (the one Tim and I dusted two days ago) a token; "dog tags" on a metal chain. One tag says, 'diabetes,' the other 'Medic Alert.' They're old; the symbols are ones not used during any recent decade. When I touch it, it vibrates in my hand. Tim and I stare at one another in silent astonishment. I'm not crazy. The spirits were listening to me.

Back on my steps in the back yard I ache for another deep experience like this and others I've had. I believe they will somehow shore up my belief and soothe my suspicion that I'm dreaming it all.

It's a struggle some days to maintain my faith, especially on days when my fifty-year-old friend who also works as a professional energy medicine practitioner, calls to tell me she's had a recurrence of ovarian cancer. Her chance of survival is less than 10%. Soberly I ask myself, God, Source, whoever is listening in the vast universe, *What's the purpose, what's the growth and healing of that?* I want to scream and rage and break something. No, it isn't always easy. I'm human. I hurt. I have fears. Finding deeper meaning in the stories can sometimes feel like I'm putting ice cream over poop.

And then, as I center myself after my emotional flood, I'm balanced into my faith again. The more I speak my truth, whether it is the voice of my uncertainty or the voice of my Soul, the more I am able to experience my wholeness, my Divine Sovereignty. Divine Sovereignty is the part of me that's free. When I feel my Divine Sovereignty I know I have dominion over my life in so much as I feel connected to the Greater Plan and that I have a voice. Instead of feeling like a pawn in a game, my Divine Sovereignty has power, wisdom, and the ability to choose my destiny.

Destiny is determined not by fate or luck or bad luck or favor; it's determined by the choices we make. The choices we make are determined by how we heal the traumatic stories of our lives. I choose love, compassion, forgiveness, joy, optimism because of my decision to find blessings wrapped within my sometimes catastrophic, sometimes merely troubling, stories.

It's easy to choose trust and passion, joy and love when what we are experiencing is inviting, comfortable, and is everything we want. The real test of destiny is if we can find love in the face of bitterness, if we can find compassion in the midst of hostility, if we can find hope when heartache surrounds us. If we can do that, then, and only then, do we have Divine Sovereignty.

An important step of healing is to find a reality beyond the pain living in our traumatic stories. To expand our awareness of life, we have to remember *we are more than our story*, more than the pain within our story. So long as we remain centered in the heartache, the tragedy, the pain, all we can taste, all we can hear and feel, is suffering and grief. With effort, we can deliberately choose to reach outside the anguish and expand our reality. When we do, the pain is just as important; it is still just as big, but it doesn't fill all of us. Our hundred pounds of pain is still a hundred pounds. Instead of trying to fit it all in a teacup, when we remember we are more than the misery of our story, we have all of heaven and earth in which to carry it. There is available space for healing to begin.

This acceptance is far different from denial or positive thinking. Those are coping strategies that do not honor the truth of the situation. Honoring the truth, healing (or understanding) the fear and grief is a quantum step over a thin line. Most people believe they are doing good to think positive thoughts that override any negative thoughts.

Superficially this is true. But a far more powerful and authentic and healthful way to be is to own the wicked, ugly, frightening, and agonizing truth while simultaneously choosing optimism. So the mantra becomes, "Even though I'm being treated for cancer now, I'm strong and healthy." Or, "I have judgments and biases, but I am not my judgments." It takes a lot of consciousness training to know if we are authentically embracing our Divine Sovereignty or if we are using our well-developed coping strategies.

I've missed opportunities to extend my heart and I've neglected my soul in exchange for mocha lattes, unnecessary handbags, and other human indulgences. Some days I'm strong and life is comfortable. And other days there's a stone in my shoe. I've learned to embrace the imperfections in me and in every person and in every relationship.

As I close my own story, I invite you to consider opening your story to find healing and blessings waiting patiently to be unearthed. As you do, remember that there are some life events that we never get over. The best we can do is to integrate our most profound losses. Although the injustice is great and the grief consuming, you can transform the gash into a scar. Death that comes too early, wicked abuse, loss that remains forever, like blindness, will leave an indelible mark.

One of the difficulties in coping with grief and loss is that after time, people expect us to have "moved on" and to be finished with our mourning. Wrong. Anniversary dates, holidays, and special occasions can and will revive the sorrow as though the loss were happening in the present moment. When you get a phone call from a grieving friend be open, listen, and invite the bereaved into your hands and heart. Rejection, avoidance, and lack of compassion make an already torturous memory more painful. Don't try to fix your friend by making suggestions for how she can feel better or try to re-direct her thoughts. This is disrespectful and is seldom the help he is seeking. Be understanding, be tolerant, listen, offer words of understanding, admit your inability to stop the pain for her, tell him "I wish this weren't so hard, but it makes sense to me how you feel."

When your own grief reawakens, respect yourself and your emotions. Allow them to come forward and reach out without shame if that's what you need.

Your healing will arrive during the darkness. It will come quietly and gently when you're not expecting it. No matter what path of self-discovery, self-awareness, or healing you choose, come to it gradually and in reverence for the story of your life, for the upheaval and for the ecstasy that has paved the roadway that has brought you "here." If you can do nothing else, just breathe. All of us who have traveled a path of healing, who have wrestled with the beast and the angel within, know that we matter and that our salvation was worth everything it took to discover our living Souls, and the same is true for you. You have Beings beside you who will never leave you. If you only realized all of the heavenly entities who are at your side, at this moment, you would never, ever be afraid again.

Above all else, remain faithful in your faith.

I believe I came to this earth as a soul and took on a body. I believe we all do. I have soul-work to do while I'm in this body.

In 2009 my stepdaughter, Bethany, gave birth to our first grandchild, Ayden Miya. Ayden lived less than three weeks, and I believe she did the soul work she was meant to do in her brief, earthly life. I wrote a story about her and gave it to Bethany. I described Ayden's birth and I believe that my own birth was similar. I see it happening like this:

"A drop of rose-colored dew is released from the hand of the Divine, falling to earth from a moonbeam in the deep, dark blue sky of an early summer evening. The dewdrop whirled on her shimmering crystal line, finally cascading into a pool of azure water covered in opalescent jewels.

She brought with her hundreds of lessons to learn, tens of dozens of stories to live, a bank full of tears to shed, and countless opportunities to laugh and love."

I'm going to live intensely, with all that I have. I'm committed to do the work of my Soul while I'm here. I'm going to keep death close to me, so I remember—remember to tell people I love them, remember not to waste a single moment, remember to use my time here for living and not for mourning more than is necessary. I'm going to find reasons to feel awe on an ordinary day. I'm going to live my life shamelessly loving the things I love: beautiful clothing, beautiful spaces, beautiful food and beautiful nature because beauty is healing. I'm going to continue to heal myself and to do my best to assist others in their own healing. I'm going to use my life for good so that after I'm gone, the universe does not regret me.

When the time comes for me to return to my original home, I imagine I will gather myself into a tiny pulsing ball of pure golden light, just as Ayden did. I will welcome my rest after my work on this earth is done. I will glide peacefully into the center of the azure pool. Here, I will be held by the caressing waters where I can dream, and refresh, and consider my next plan. When the moment is right, I, as a golden ball of light, will rise confidently and fearlessly above the surface of the pool.

And then I imagine a shimmering golden veil will drop from the heavens. As the veil ever so gently dips into the blue pool, I, the golden drop of light, will willingly reunite with this magnificent veil of ecstatic presence. I will weave myself into the veil, tucking myself safely and snugly into a tiny place that is missing one radiant thread. When I do, the veil will silently lift itself higher and higher into the dawning day. From earth, the golden veil will appear as emerging beams of sunlight cresting above the horizon.

Finally, as I ride in the golden veil, completing my reunion with the sun and the entire cosmos, majestic colors of purple and orange and pink will seep into the sky. This will be my face for eternity. And what I will feel is triumphant glory, unspeakable ease, and a reunion with a love so great, so unconditional, I will realize that I have wanted this moment since I first drew breath.

And so it is.

Love, Shelli

"Who could ask for anything more?"

Irving Berlin

*"My Soul is from elsewhere; I'm sure of that.
One day I will return to that place"*

Rumi

*"Don't ask yourself what the world needs. Ask yourself what
makes you come alive, and then go and do that. Because
what the world needs is people who have come alive."*

Harold Whitman

*"When you come to the edge of all you know you must
believe in one of two things:
there will be ground to stand on.
Or, you will be given wings to fly."*

Unknown

*"Give thanks or go home a waste of spark. Speak, or let
the maker take back your throat. March, or let the creator
rescind your feet. Dream, or let your god destroy your good
and fertile mind. This is your warning; this, your birthright.
Do not let the universe regret you."*

Marty Mc Donnell

ABOUT THE AUTHOR

SHELLI AND HER HUSBAND, BRENT NELSON, LIVE IN BLOOMINGTON, Minnesota near the beautiful Minnesota River valley. They have one daughter, Bethany Nelson. Their current four-legged child is Meadowlawn Kennel's Dancing the Jig, aka Lindi.

Shelli enjoys the outdoors and gardening. She and Brent enjoy entertaining, home renovation, and interior design. They are passionate about healthy food and healthy living.

Shelli founded Rukha® Academy of Healing Arts and Science in 2009. She is the acting Vice-President and Brent is the President of the school. Rukha® Academy is licensed under the Minnesota Department of Higher Education. The professional curriculum provides education in energy medicine and transpersonal psychology.

For information about Rukha® Academy of Healing Arts and Science, visit

www.RukhaAcademy.com

For information about Shelli's healing practice, Healing Professionals, LLC, visit:

www.HealingProfessionals.com

www.ShelliStangerNelson.com

For information about diabetes support and management in the USA, visit:

www.Diabetes.org

CPSIA information can be obtained
at www.ICGtesting.com
Printed in the USA
FFOW05n0122280117